MY CHILD, DIABETES AND ME

Despina Margiori

MY CHILD, DIABETES, AND ME

A personal account of our symbiosis with type one diabetes (and celiac disease)

First published in Greek November 2014 under the title: „Το Παιδί μου, ο Διαβήτης κι Εγώ. Μία προσωπική μαρτυρία για την διαβίωσή μας με τον διαβήτη τύπου 1"

Translated from Greek by Despina Margiori

Edited by Zoe Swenson-Wright

DEDICATION

For Danái and Ióli, and for all type one diabetic
children

PRAISE FOR THE GREEK EDITION

"I read it twice and it is amazing"

R. Lagiou (The first woman in Greece who used an insulin pump)

"The book of Despina Margiori, a garden of sentiments and teachings, will travel – translated – around the world"

E. Delidaki (Medical Journalist)

"A while ago I electronically 'fell over' this unique, amazing, guide book of Mrs Despina Margiori. A life lesson, this so well written and at the same time authentic book will stay in your mind and with you for a long time after you finish reading it..."

R. Stratila (Blogger: sugar mama)

"Bravo. Any effort to teach is beneficial"

N. Valvis (Medical doctor, endocrinologist, diabetic type one)

"A book to be read by everyone: Doctors, patients, and non- patients"

M. Prokopiou (Medical doctor, endocrinologist)

"I did not get on my bus because I did not want to stop reading it! I kept reading the whole night..."

E. Vlachou (Children hairdresser, with a type two diabetic in the family)

"Despina Margiori's MY CHILD, DIABETES AND ME: A hymn to endeavor"

K. Brotzaki (reader)

"A useful tool for informing the parents and the children of the schools we serve!"

V. Vasileiou (teacher)

"A nice way to inform children, parents, and teachers. We thank you a lot"

E. Moutsiouli (teacher)

"The whole family read it and it helped us a lot. Thank you for all you do for us"

Anonymous (retired teacher, grandfather of a five year old type one diabetic girl)

"Every so often I would grab the phone and call my partner at work and read to him what in the book really touched me. At the end he asked me to buy one more

book to give to one of his customers who has two diabetic children…. This book helped me with MY issues!"

M. Dimaki (beautician)

TABLE OF CONTENTS

PREFACE

Five years ago our life took an unexpected turn. The older of my two daughters was diagnosed with diabetes type one, suddenly and without any warning signs. She was then eight years old. As is well known, type one diabetes has a permanent character and is treated either through the use of multiple, daily insulin injections or by using an insulin pump.

During these past five years, my daughter and I, as well as the rest of the family, have experienced a tsunami of feelings and many demanding situations. The power they exercised over us, as well as the changes they brought to our lives during the first few minutes, days, and months of living with diabetes, convinced me that these experiences would have a permanent impact. I believed that they would weigh down our future in the same shattering way they did in the beginning, regardless of the passage of years. Back then, at the beginning of our symbiosis with type one diabetes, I felt as if despair, bitterness, fear, and insecurity would accompany me with the same intensity and frequency for the rest of my life, mutilating all of my energy and enthusiasm for living.

It has not been like that. The diagnosis has affected every member of the family. The experiences we gained through this sudden change of direction—as well as the feelings they aroused—are described in this book. I naturally present my own feelings and observations and my interpretations of the feelings of my diabetic daughter because I am in a position to describe them with absolute precision and can vouch for their honest and authentic character. For this reason, the description of our life with diabetes is a subjective one. Since my younger daughter also had to deal with the tensions and changes caused by diabetes, I have also described—even if not extensively—the impact of this all had on her.

My purpose in recounting and publishing these personal experiences has been complex. Through writing this book, past situations rose to the surface and into my consciousness. This enabled me to remember feelings and to become aware of the psychological changes taking place within me. Looking back over the past made me see clearly where I started from and how far I travelled in the five years after my child's diagnosis.

By writing this book, I undertook an intensive process of self-observation. Looking back over everything that has happened and remembering details and situations has helped me put valuable experiences in order. It has given me a chance to devote time to them—time that they deserved—and to recognize how they partially changed my priorities and interests. Revisiting the past has had a liberating, cathartic effect. It has made me realize that these experiences made a valuable contribution to my further psychological maturation and development, enabling me to constructively support my children.

Despite all this, my biggest motivation in writing this book has been the need I felt, over an extended period of time, to help other parents of diabetic children—and especially the mothers of such children. I wanted to help them face the challenges and problems of life with diabetes type one with strength and optimism. I have met many mothers of type one diabetic children who do not seem to have found a way to accept their children's condition, despite the passage of a significant amount of time since diagnosis. I have met mothers who have not found a way out of the sorrow they feel, and others who don't dare to look reality straight in the eyes, perhaps because they are afraid of experiencing more pain than they can bear.

At the same time, I have learned that mothers do not always seek help when they need it. They remain alone in a tortuous world of negative emotions, unable to escape from damaging ways of thinking. Across many nationalities, these women have made me believe that many mothers of diabetic children are looking for a guide, someone able to stand up for them and comprehend their

pain. They have made me understand their need to hear hopeful, consoling words from someone living in the same world and facing the same problems. When I meet other mothers of diabetic children, I realize how much we all long to hear alternative ways of thinking about life with diabetes, in order to gain strength and move on with our lives.

I hope that this book will reach mothers of children who have just been diagnosed with type one diabetes. Perhaps reading about my experiences will encourage these women and help them get through the tremendously demanding first hours with diabetes, so that they will not be as scared as I was back then, during my first contact with the condition. This book is also for mothers of the future, those who do not yet know that they will be entering our world, the world of diabetes.

Sharing with readers the valuable knowledge I acquired through the process of coming to terms with my daughter's diagnosis is my way of trying to ease the psychological pain so widely felt in the diabetic world. If this book can help in any way to decrease the agony and fear caused by a child's diagnosis of type one diabetes, then I will have achieved my goal. Even without knowing the readers of this book personally, I feel an absolute understanding of and compassion for any parent whose child is diagnosed with type one diabetes. I am sharing my knowledge and experiences with unknown readers in the hope of improving their quality of life. I want all who live with and care for diabetic children to realize that your life does not stop when diabetes rudely and abruptly invades it.

Through this book, I also appeal to non-sufferers, to all of the groups of people who make up, in different ways, the social environment of the diabetic child. I appeal to the non-diabetic world to become more aware of the special needs of diabetic families. This book addresses medical staff, teachers, relatives, friends, and neighbors—all who witness the adversities of families of diabetic children on a daily basis. In this way, I hope to sensitize international society to the ways in which we all think about and treat people with special needs—people who must try harder than others to survive. I appeal to everyone to reach out to those who are daily confronted with physical and psychological pain, and to those who must constantly battle diabetes. I hope to encourage all of us to stop and listen carefully to the lessons of life offered by individuals forced to live in extraordinary ways.

As I was driving today on a narrow, curving road, going uphill and downhill, it occurred to me that in order to get the best performance from the engine of my car, I needed to turn down the radio (a song I was enjoying) so that I could hear the engine and judge when to change gears. I realized that this was how all human beings should interact. Helping other people function as well as possible when coping with a difficult situation requires being willing to listen to what we are being told, and adjusting our words and deeds accordingly.

It is my hope that this book will motivate people who do not live with the challenges of type one diabetes, regardless of their social roles, to turn down their own mental soundtracks and make a sincere effort to understand the problems of diabetic children and their families. By understanding the many hardships that these children are confronted with, others can help to alleviate their pain.

I could never have written this book (whatever my own personal needs) without the consent of my diabetic daughter, Danai, the main protagonist of this narrative. I thank her immensely for her generosity, and for her willingness to allow her story to be used to help others achieve a better symbiosis with type one diabetes. Her decision to do this has been precious. Perhaps this account will motivate her, sometime in the future, to explore her own past experiences. Perhaps it will awaken the need in her to describe and interpret the way her feelings have evolved since the day when so much changed for her so suddenly.

I want to thank both my daughters, Danai and Ioli, and my husband for the moral support I received when writing this book. By demonstrating their faith in me, they helped this dream become reality. I thank my daughters for all the times they closed the door of my office and let me continue writing. I thank them for their tender kisses and warm hugs, for the hot tea they brought me and the meals they cooked, for their belief that this book deserved to go out into the world, and most of all for understanding how precious this piece of work was for me.

Recently we visited a museum in Berlin where anyone could write a wish on a pomegranate-shaped piece of paper and hang it on a tree. Danai wrote: "I want my mother´s book to become a best-seller," this time giving her written consent to my decision to share aspects of our family life.

I would like to express my gratitude to Zoe Swenson-Wright for the patience she demonstrated answering my questions each time we worked on the book!

In order to respect their right to anonymity, all of the people mentioned in this book, who are not members of my family, have been given fictitious names. However, both of my daughters have chosen to be referred to by their real names.

My purpose and hope is to speak to the world as a mother, using the direct language of the heart.

With love,

Despina Margiori

1. THE LAST FEW MINUTES BEFORE DIABETES

That Monday afternoon in the pediatrician's office was the last time Danai and I ever played hangman without the shadow of diabetes. We were waiting for her to be examined by a doctor who had been her pediatrician since birth and who knew her very well. His office waiting room was well-equipped with toys to keep children busy, but Danai, who was eight years old, always found hangman more challenging and amusing, especially because she could write very good Greek, despite having been born in Germany, where we live.

With no suspicion of what was to follow a few minutes later, and no idea that all of our lives (not only Danai's but those of her parents and sister) were about to change, she and I found a piece of chalk. With cunning smiles on our faces, we teased, "I'll give you a difficult one, see if you can get it," and began to draw on the blackboard. In our other hands, we held thick, wet, yellow sponges, ready to erase anything we didn't want to see anymore. That wasn't like real life. Life doesn't provide any kind of sponge to erase what you don't want to see.

On Mondays, most private doctors' offices are filled with patients. We were used to this pattern. It happens because many people's bodies, including the bodies of children, seem to relax and show symptoms of weakness when the weekend arrives. In the majority of cases, it is nothing serious—perhaps a common illness, which can wait until Monday, when a doctor you trust can provide treatment.

That Monday, however, we were waiting in the pediatrician's office for a different reason. The previous Friday, Danai had come home from school with a message from the principal, who also happened to be her sports teacher, suggesting that she be examined by her doctor as soon as possible. He had noticed Danai getting very tired during her swimming class.

This teacher and gymnast's experience, observation skills, and sense of responsibility sent us to the doctor. We would never have guessed that Danai needed medical help, even if we had noticed that she was getting tired too easily in the swimming pool. She had always been very good at sports and had never had trouble with any physical activity. Later, we would be asked many times by different people whether Danai was drinking an excessive amount of water at night, whether she was losing weight despite eating a normal diet, and whether she needed the toilet too often. The answer to all of these questions was no.

So this is why Danai and I were playing hangman without the slightest suspicion that anything was wrong with her. We were sure that the doctor would carry out a routine examination and tell us he could not see anything unusual happening in Danai's body. I felt sure that my daughter was healthy. If she got tired when she was swimming, surely that just reflected her physical condition on a particular day. That Monday, we were still laughing, writing, and erasing words from the blackboard without any worries about possible future scenarios.

Until that Monday afternoon, we lived a predictable life. The children were growing and needed new clothes and shoes. They had play dates with friends; we organized trips abroad and out to the countryside. We shared meals without thinking about exactly how much food to consume at which precise times. We played with balls and on trampolines. We cycled as

much as we wanted whenever we felt like it. We baked cakes, had picnics, visited zoos and museums, played board games, and read children's books. We built snowmen, watched children's movies, invited friends home, and spent endless hours in playgrounds, bookshops, and swimming pools. The children lived and played happily, as young children should. I enjoyed all this with a constant, and perhaps unconscious, sense of indescribable joy and gratitude for the privilege of motherhood.

So that Monday, I was playing hangman with a deep sense of satisfaction about the point I had reached my life. I felt reassured that everything was the way I wanted it to be. Every morning, when I woke up, this sense of satisfaction gave me the strength and energy I needed to face any routine challenge. I was full of ideas about how to bring up my children, as well as plans and ambitions about my own life and career.

The pediatrician's waiting room was getting emptier as Danai and I filled up the blackboard with lines, letters, and the funny heads and deformed bodies of those being hanged for choosing the wrong letters— over and over again, until the word one of us had thought up for the other was finally revealed. This moment is imprinted on my memory forever because of what happened only minutes later. I cannot forget how spontaneously and affectionately we laughed when we managed to figure out a riddle and rescue the chalk figure on the blackboard from hanging. I cannot forget how calm and relaxed we felt as the minutes passed.

We had to wait a long time because the pediatrician had made an extra appointment for us and had many other extra appointments that day. Ioli, my other daughter, had gone to a friend's house because sitting in the waiting room would have exhausted her. She was only five. I was planning to pick her up on the way home, as we usually did. My husband was abroad on a business trip.

At last we had played long enough and were wondering when it would finally be Danai's turn to be examined. We sat together, giving each other energy and hoping for a quick appointment so that we could go home. When the doctor's assistant opened the door and called Danai's name, we stood up eagerly, relieved that our turn had come. We collected our stuff and followed the assistant, feeling perfectly relaxed, both physically and mentally. We had visited this office several times before, mainly for required, routine examinations and vaccinations or to be treated for some minor disease. We were accustomed to the ritual of visiting the pediatrician; both my daughters had done this many times without experiencing any psychological trauma.

The doctor's office consisted of three examination rooms. We did not usually use the room his assistant directed us to that day. It was the smallest of the three, and I guessed that other children must be using the two larger rooms. I was wrong; this room contained cardiogram equipment. As soon as he heard the reason for our visit, Danai's doctor thought she would need a cardiogram test.

I remember standing next to Danai, who was now lying down with suction cups stuck to her body and cables hanging in all directions. I smiled at her reassuringly—a Mom's smile (bestowed by the person who always knows best), promising that this was nothing serious and everything would turn out fine. I was her Mom and Danai trusted me to do everything

under the sun to protect her and her sister; she knew I would do whatever it took to keep her healthy and happy. My smile and a few jokes in Greek that only Danai could understand made her relax and feel unafraid of the cardiogram. She lay still until we could hear the sound of printing, with the ink jumping up and down on white paper, declaring that Danai's tiredness during swimming had nothing to do with her heart.

"See, Danai?" I reassured her. "I told you it was nothing!" I remember saying that while the assistant was still removing the suction cups and cables from my daughter's eight-year-old body. Danai trusted me and her face was calm. Eight years of personal experience had taught her that the woman standing beside her, as she lay waiting for the doctor, had been there since the day she was born and knew what she was talking about.

We heard movement and waited for the ever-polite and busy pediatrician, Dr. P., to make a quick visit, on his way to examining another child. We were sure he would tell us, with his usual lightning speed that Danai seemed to have no problem: the tiredness her teacher had noticed at the swimming pool was nothing serious—Danai could get dressed and go home. This is what we expected and wanted to hear. So when Dr. P. opened the door and made his usual quick entrance, Danai and I immediately started looking for her clothes and my bag. We stood by the door, eager to say goodbye and leave the room free for the next child, who would also be hoping to go home or to the playground as fast as possible.

This time, however, our automatic response was interrupted, because the doctor could not let Danai go before examining her urine. No problem. It's easy to give a urine sample to exclude a bladder infection, I thought. Even then, Danai and I were certain that good old Dr. P., whom we'd trusted for many years, just wanted to make sure that she was fine before letting us leave to pick up Ioli from her friend's house and go home to live the way we always had.

Dr. P's assistant took the urine sample away to test it. Up to that point I remember the blood in my veins flowing unnoticed. I was calm and pleased with the fact that we had such good medical care to keep our children healthy. I remember feeling sure that Danai was fine.

Looking back now, I wonder why I rushed, that Monday morning, to make her the earliest possible appointment with the pediatrician. What made me drive Danai there after school, if I was so sure my daughter was fine? Why, that afternoon, did I ignore the fact that she had her regular, scheduled Monday dance class, which, for years, she had only missed when she was sick? Why did I ignore my husband's advice, who pointed out, before leaving for London, that Monday afternoon wasn't a good time to take Danai to the doctor because it clashed with her dance class, which was already paid for? What made me hurry to ask the doctor's opinion, when I believed that my daughter was fine?

Five years have passed since the moment when the pediatrician's assistant entered the examination room, holding Danai's urine test results. Earlier that day, I had chatted to this woman about her personal life. She told me that she had decided to quit her job and start selling sausages in a canteen. She wanted to be self-employed and was tired of working in a private doctor's office. I remember feeling sad about her decision, as I'd known her for years and liked her. I did not know that the sadness to come would be far bigger and longer-lasting.

2. THE FIRST SUSPICIONS

The expression on the face of the doctor's assistant changed as she entered the room. I have always observed the people around me carefully, especially the people I talk to. Something had certainly changed in her facial expression, and I knew it had nothing to do with her decision to change jobs. I knew she was experienced enough to understand a urine test and did not need the doctor's medical expertise to become alarmed or realize that something was wrong with this child. I started to feel intensely the blood in my veins, the disturbing beating of my heart, and the sweat in my palms, although the room was air-conditioned. At that moment, Dr. P. entered the room hurriedly. He sat down quickly in front of his computer and his assistant said the first words that would change Danai's future and that of our family: "the color"—the color of the tape she had used for Danai's urine test was suspiciously dark, the first indication that something was wrong. I turned and looked at it. It was dark green.

The next set of visual stimuli I perceived came from the familiar face of my daughter's doctor. Never before, in eight years of working in partnership with this man, had I ever seen what I saw then—an expression that still makes me feel the way I felt then, even five years later. Agony, fear, desperation, and denial conquered me. My survival mechanism prompted me to become defensive as quickly as possible. I did not want the doctor to tell me anything alarming about my child; I did not want any more time to pass. I wanted to remain in the same joyful, carefree state of mind I'd been in while playing hangman in the waiting room with this child I'd given birth to, who had made me appreciate what real happiness was. All this I felt in a fraction of a second, while the doctor turned and looked at his assistant, who would leave her job in a few days and make a new start, far away from urine tests and mothers drowning in tears and fear.

Danai was sitting down. So was the doctor. More stimuli were hammering at my senses. This time, they were audible. The doctor's voice sounded like drumming when he asked, with unprecedented seriousness and soberness, what Danai had had for lunch before coming to his office. I could tell by how quickly he asked one question after another that Danai's case was serious. I found a chair and sat down too. I felt that, no matter how much I loved my daughter and wanted to protect her, just now I had to sit down, so as not to collapse in the middle of this small room filled with medical equipment. I understood where all of this was heading. He was hinting that there were high levels of sugar in my daughter's blood.

Danai had not wanted much lunch that day. She had eaten only a boiled potato and some boiled corn. Did she drink anything other than water? No. This was what the doctor wanted to know and what I told him. Danai had been to school that day and would normally be hungry. But her body knew better. She could not eat much, because her body couldn't supply the right amount of insulin to handle larger quantities of food. Her own body knew what it needed—I was the one who didn't. The doctor asked question after question with remarkable persistence, his face expressing considerable anxiety. However, my psychological state prevented me from hearing the actual sound of his voice. I could not bear to see the worry on his face as he asked what my eight-year-old had eaten for lunch—the child who was now sitting next to me trying to understand what was happening, the child I adored and wanted to protect from every kind of harm.

During the course of a few minutes, my role changed. The mother-protector, the mother-pacifier, the supportive, smiling mother, the funny, inventive woman could no longer tell her daughter that she was well and everything would be fine, that it was nothing serious and there wouldn't be any pain. Suddenly, without any warning, I felt my power decreasing. I felt my ability to protect my daughter diminishing. Without being asked whether I wanted my role to fall to a different level (that of a woman needing help to support her child), I felt myself losing the power to protect Danai or to shield her from situations that could threaten her physical and mental integrity. I felt I was losing my own arms and could no longer hug my child and help her escape the lurking danger entering our lives.

Danai could not understand what was causing so much turmoil, in this little room, between two adults she absolutely trusted. She did not understand, but I did. Dr. P. was not asking in a casual, meaningless way (in fact, he was almost shouting) how much of what kind of food Danai had eaten for lunch. His urgency, as he told me to take her to the hospital immediately, was no accident. There was a sense of high alarm everywhere. From that point on, everything happened very fast. A blood test followed the urine test; the results showed that Danai's case was really an emergency.

I could not control my physical reactions any more, no matter how much I wanted to keep my child from worrying. I was shivering and crying, and telling the doctor that what was happening was not fair, that I had breastfed my daughter for the first year of her life and always took good care of her nutritional needs. The doctor knew us well, and agreed with everything I said. He offered to call an ambulance to transport us immediately to the hospital, since I seemed unable to drive.

Now Danai started crying. She understood that something was wrong with her, without knowing exactly what it was. I remember her face full of tears, as she told me she didn't want to go to the hospital in an ambulance. I could hardly refuse to take her there—there was nothing I wouldn't do to make this emergency less upsetting for her. However, I was now a different person from the relaxed, calm mother who'd felt so happy about finding a parking space just outside the doctor's office, a few hours before our introduction to the world of diabetes type one.

I told the doctor that I would drive Danai to the hospital myself, whatever shape I was in, and he accepted that.

Dr. P. asked me not to go home, although our house was only a five-minute drive from his office and a three-minute drive from the hospital. I told him that

I had to make two urgent phone calls: one to my husband in London, to let him know how lucky it was that Danai had missed her dance class, because she urgently needed to go to the hospital. The other phone call was about Ioli, who was expecting to be picked up from her friend's house soon, so that she, Danai, and I could all go home together. I had to tell my friend that five-year-old Ioli would need to spend the night with her, and that Ioli's Dad was on his way home. I hoped my younger daughter wouldn't think her whole family had vanished suddenly and unexpectedly.

The doctor asked for my cell phone number before we left his office and I gave it to him. He wished me courage and let us go devastated, crying, worrying, upset, and uncertain about what would happen next. From that point on, I felt immensely empty, defeated and torn in pieces. However, more than ever, Danai needed me to be strong and soothing. Out of love for her, I found some residual mental strength and used it to calm her down.

"What does 'diabetes' mean?" eight-year-old Danai wanted to know, on our way home.

"They will tell us in the hospital," I said, hoping to avoid upsetting her even more.

Yes, we drove home and not directly to the hospital. This one time, I did not follow the doctor's advice—partly because we needed to grab a few things from home to survive our first night in the hospital, and partly because I wanted to make sure that my five-year-old daughter had what she needed to stay overnight at the neighbor's. Ioli was still playing there, carefree—waiting for me to show up so she could jump into my arms, smiling and ready to go home.

Everything happened very fast. We climbed up the stairs in our four-story building, and then left our apartment with tears in our eyes. The travelling bag we always took on excursions was transformed into a hospital bag. I gave our apartment key to the woman Ioli was spending the night with. She met me out on the street so that my younger daughter wouldn't see me and want to come too. At least if she had a key to our house, my friend could get everything Ioli needed for the night: her nightgown, toothpaste, toothbrush, and Sakis—the toy rabbit she always slept with. I could not do anything more for her because we had to rush to the hospital.

There, we were already expected. Our pediatrician had called the children's hospital diabetes ward and a room was ready for us. The first tests though took place on the ground floor of the hospital, minutes after we arrived. We were met by a Greek doctor, a friend of ours, who happened to be working there. She found Danai and me plumped down on the couch in the hospital reception area—distraught, hugging each other, and waiting for a nurse to come tell us what to do. Our friend had been asked to receive a new patient into the diabetes ward and had recognized Danai's name.

The day before, this friend had visited us at home and played with the children. I had told her that I was taking Danai to the doctor for tests, on her teacher's advice, but none of us imagined the circumstances under which we would meet again, just twenty-four hours later. At that moment, in the hospital reception area, I felt physically and mentally numb—forced into a kind of paralysis. I did not want to know; I did not want to hear; I did not want to think about or accept the situation we had suddenly found ourselves in. My psyche was protesting against this enormous betrayal.

This is how our Greek doctor-friend found us. She called to me from a distance, and approached looking visibly worried. Danai showed no hint of her usual vivaciousness and spontaneity. In the past, whenever this friend visited, Danai was always up to some mischief—joking and laughing and full of hairdressing ideas that she demonstrated using our friend's head. Such moments now belonged to the past. Our old friend was dressed in a white gown and had come to escort us to the diabetes ward—the scenario now unrolling

seemed completely cut off from our time spent with her at home. Danai waited in silence. She had me beside her and felt safe, but her eyes were full of tears.

As we followed our friend, she told us what would happen next. She would insert a catheter under Danai's skin, a standard procedure for all children admitted to this hospital. In a small, white, unadorned room, I watched the young doctor's hands shake as she tried to pierce my child's hand. She knows Danai so well, I thought, and never expected to have to admit her to the diabetes department. The needle went under her skin, together with a small catheter. It was Danai's first experience of the physical pain caused by diabetes.

Nobody wants to feel physical or any other kind of pain. Once again, I had to play my role and be the encouraging Mom—the comforter and strong woman Danai always looked to in times of despair. However, my own body and soul were collapsing just when I was needed most. Tension and the constant changes to our reality were taking a toll. This change would be with me long into the future; at that moment, however, there was no time to speculate or imagine.

What will happen next? What do we have to do now? Where do we have to go? Who do we have to talk to? The minutes were passing like hours, and the hours were passing like months. Anxiety, fear, and a touch of hope (perhaps someone had made a mistake?)

confused my consciousness, making me feel like a leaf blown in the wind. I was able to walk and wanted to support and reassure Danai, who was looking to me for some kind of guidance or advice that would make her immediate future predictable. I told her not to worry—they would tell us what to do. That was all. I couldn't offer her anything more than encouragement, to help her stay calm for the next few minutes. Danai remained worried, but she did stay calm.

Our friend escorted us to the diabetes ward, where we would spend the first night. The days were short and it was getting dark; tomorrow would be the first day of September, bringing with it a new life for us. We oriented ourselves in the new room. Here is the toilet and over there is the shower. Here is a bed with remote control and there is the view from the window. I felt quietness, absolute insecurity, and a continuing numbness. The first nurse arrived to measure the sugar levels in Danai´s blood. This time, she used the diabetes ward's measuring equipment, an instrument that looked like an oversized remote control. From now on, everything would have to be recorded in detail. The measurements continued all through the night, each and every hour. At first, the indications were unclear, and the doctors could not diagnose Danai's condition with certainty. Her sugar levels showed significant fluctuations throughout the night. They had to wait and measure. We had to wait and worry.

I contacted the friend looking after my younger daughter, afraid that Ioli too might be feeling pain and insecurity, after being taken away so suddenly from her home environment. My friend reassured me that Ioli was sleeping. That was a relief and, for a moment, I felt slightly calmer. I could not have handled knowing that Ioli was upset because I hadn't come to take her home. I told my friend that my husband was on his way and would come straight from the airport to check on her. Danai was also sleeping, but in a hospital bed with white sheets. Despite missing the familiar colors and smells of home, she had no choice but to do

so. She was exhausted. At least my presence was helping her leave behind the worries and fears of the most demanding day of her life so far, and enabling her to sleep.

Each time the nurse came, she disinfected a patch of skin on Danai's finger and pierced it, using a diabetes test strip to absorb a drop of blood. Then she announced a number and immediately left the room in the same impersonal way she had entered it. Whenever she did this, I felt even more insecure and alone. Obviously, Danai wasn't the first child whose blood sugar levels this nurse had measured. She carried out her routine, not stopping to consider that it was our first night in the diabetes ward. Danai went on sleeping. That was good, I thought—at least she wasn't feeling the prolonged agony of waiting for a result or diagnosis.

Time passed extremely slowly. The measuring of Danai's blood sugar levels went on and on. Nobody could give us a clear picture of what would happen next. Fatigue was muddled with exhaustion, exhaustion with a secret hope that perhaps there had been some mistake. All my thoughts were clouded with sorrow. This confusion was intensified by the doctor on duty during the first hours of that September night. She emerged suddenly out of the semi-lit corridor of the diabetes department, asking to talk to me and my husband, who had returned from his trip and was now in the ward.

Her words cut through the quietness of the night. They were savage—the hardest, most unnerving, inhuman and devastating words for mind or body that I had ever heard. The doctors had decided that Danai should have a special test that morning so that they could reach a conclusion. "But," said this white figure, standing alone in the middle of the empty hospital corridor—apparently without the slightest suspicion of the impact of what she was saying was having on me— "you should already start preparing for the result. Everything indicates that it's diabetes type one." She said this, and then disappeared into the darkness, just as she had emerged from it.

No, I thought. I will not accept that. I cannot and I do not want to. This is about my daughter. I was the one who gave birth to her, not that lady in white who believes she can enter our lives so abruptly and speak in such a harsh way about something she learned from books, which we now have to begin living with. Diabetes was threatening to penetrate our existence, dominate our lives, become real, and determine everything. No. Perhaps this is all a mistake. Perhaps it was a mistake that our pediatrician sent us to the hospital in such a hurry. Perhaps it was a mistake that they stuck needles into Danai's fingers so many times, hurting her when she could not defend herself. The whole of yesterday was wrong; the whole night has been wrong; everybody has been wrong. Let's just hope that's true. Just tell me that you've made mistakes, so that I can feel strong again, pack up our stuff, and take my child home from the hospital in the morning. Let me pick up my other child and get her ready for kindergarten. Let Danai go to school tomorrow. She is so young! Let her laugh and run and shout. You cannot drown our lives so suddenly and unexpectedly. Is that too much to ask? Just let us leave behind these diagnoses, tests, and possible and probable scenarios. Our familiar, daily, sweet life—I want that back.

My husband also heard the lady in white give her warning. He stood next to me speechless, clouded over with the news. He accepted the possibility that something might be wrong, but I was not convinced that anything had really changed in the body of my eight-year-old daughter, the child I cherished even before she was born. WHY? Why is this happening to me? Why to this child? Not yet. The fearful morning had not yet arrived, and the notorious sugar test that would decide everything had not yet been carried out. I was glad when the doctor disappeared down the semi-lit corridor of the diabetes ward. I did not want to hear anything more. I stood outside Danai's room and held all of these questions deep inside me. I was hurting enough as it was. I didn't want to hear anything more from anyone, unless they could tell me that my daughter was fine and everything was a mistake. I would forgive them all for their mistakes. Mistakes happen. I only needed someone to smile and tell me that everything was all right and we could go home. That was the only message I could endure. Nothing else. Danai was still sleeping and the sky was dark, like my inner world.

3. THE MOMENT OF TRUTH

I don't remember how many endless hours it took for morning to come. My senses had lost the ability to register my life passing. I just remember that it was day and Danai and I were in an examination room surrounded by hospital staff. She had swallowed some kind of liquid and her blood sugar was being measured multiple times. We had to wait a long time for the results—perhaps even hours. I don't remember exactly. I remember our Greek doctor-friend, back for a new shift, giving me some slight hope by commenting that perhaps something Danai had eaten the day before had caused all this turmoil. I remember jumping out of my chair, desperate for her to tell me that Danai was all right. Again, I had to wait for the results. They would take time.

Some hours later, our friend brought a German colleague to announce the result of the special test. I remember that it was afternoon, although my sense of time was distorted. Hours and minutes no longer mattered to me—I had learned to wait. The two women came to find me outside Danai's room, which was different from the room we had spent the night in. The corridor was lit with very disturbing lights. The moving bodies of people wandering around me, each for a different reason, were equally disturbing. Voices felt as loud as drums being played right next to me—merciless, and there to destroy my whole existence. I watched the bodies of the two doctors in white move toward me in a menacing way—steadily and rhythmically. I did not want any of this. I did not want this moment to arrive. Let's just go home, I thought. I can't take any more of this.

They both stood before me: our Greek friend who had played with my happy, lively children just two days ago and a German doctor I had never seen before. I wanted to leave. I wanted to interrupt this meeting. I couldn't stand this, and I didn't want to hear them. I longed to put my hands over my ears, close my eyes, and not hear the voices coming from the doctors' mouths or see the hurtful words their lips were forming. But the German doctor had to do her job—it's what she was paid for. At the end of her shift, she would go home. We would stay.

The results showed that my child had type one diabetes.

This second doctor coldly announced that she would be giving Danai an injection of insulin in her belly immediately! It felt as if my child was merchandise on a supermarket counter, waiting to be scanned. After all, we were in the diabetes ward and others were waiting for their doses of insulin. One more injection in another child's belly—what difference could it make to this clinical expert? Her job was to inform parents and inject their children's bellies with needles. It was not her job to clear away the rubble she left behind.

If anyone else had been there to support my daughter, I would probably have collapsed. But I was alone and had to do what I could to protect Danai from the cold hands and intentions of this doctor. If her abrupt and uncaring manner had managed to annihilate me in just a few seconds, what sort of trauma would she inflict on the eight-year-old girl lying peacefully in her hospital bed?

Our Greek friend was standing next to her colleague and trying to help with a smile. But I was shocked and sobbing—asking the diabctologist to let me talk to Danai first. I wanted to introduce the new reality in my own way, and to explain why she was still in a hospital room and could not see her friends at school. Fortunately, I convinced the doctor to delay the injection until I'd had a chance to talk to my child.

I did not stand outside her room, trying to find the right words to explain what I knew. I had not given any thought to how I might explain the situation to Danai because I was busy clinging despairingly to the life we'd had. I loved the way we lived—was it really going to end so fast? When the two doctors arrived to confirm the diagnosis, I had to talk to Danai, with or without preparation.

I had to be the one to explain to her what was happening because our relationship was based on honesty. It was important to do this quickly and fully, out of respect for her and so that she would not worry about her condition. My daughter had the right to know what was happening to her body. I had to tell her the truth because it primarily concerned her—a truth that would determine both her long- and short-term future. It was a difficult and serious truth that could not be distorted or deviated from. Somehow, I had to find the appropriate words to explain all this to an eight-year-old child without frightening her. I did not wait. I entered Danai's room quickly, also a good way for me to escape from the many disturbing stimuli in the corridor.

I found my daughter waiting, lying in bed and covered with the white hospital quilt. I could see that she wanted to know and knew I had to tell her. She asked what was going on and I couldn't put off the bad news—making her wait longer would just be more stressful. Knowing that this would be a demanding test for both of us, I started talking.

"Danai, you know how our bodies are like factories with many engines? Sometimes, some of these engines don't work the way they should and need help. It is like this with our bodies too. Organs don't always work the way they should and when that happens, we need to help them. The doctors say there's a problem with your pancreas, which is supposed to produce insulin. They say it can't make insulin on its own, so we will have to give your body insulin ourselves."

I told her the painful, hard truth and for a moment felt shocked at what I had done. Was this the right way to tell my child something so serious? Why was it that, while talking to her, I stopped feeling so much sorrow, sadness, and despair? I spoke easily, calmly, and with confidence, as if telling her that we were going to the zoo—why was that? Perhaps there is no better way to talk to a child than the way your heart dictates. Perhaps the love you feel for your child shows you what to do, even when you have to tell her that she has diabetes. At any rate, I followed my instincts when introducing Danai to her new life, and

I hope it was the right approach. In that moment, I became once again her good old, strong, and confident Mom, who knew what she was talking about.

When Danai asked how her body was going to get insulin, I had to explain. She listened to me carefully, trying to understand. She quickly realized that this was not a short-term or transient problem and became worried and upset.

"All my life I have to have injections?" was the first thing she asked, and then hid under the hospital quilt, perhaps because she did not want to hear any more. Perhaps, like me, she too wanted to escape the new reality—and the quickest way to achieve this was by going under the quilt.

I felt so much sympathy and wished that I did not have to tell her anything. I touched her with love, letting my hand rest gently on her quilt-covered body to show that I was there for her. I wanted Danai to know that diabetes would not change everything in our lives. Her mother's love would always be there to give her strength. I felt her relaxing a bit, even at this most difficult moment of her life. She carried on hiding under the hospital's borrowed sheets, which had covered who knows how many children with who knows how many problems.

"Danai, I know this is not easy for you, but you will never be alone in this. I will always be there for you," I told her, trying to do what I could to lessen her pain.

My implied promise to share the responsibility, pain, and fear, and to provide company, support, and safety eventually made her crawl out from under the covers, like a snail conquering fear and coming out of its shell.

4. TWO WEEKS OF TENSION AND INTENSIVE LESSONS

Our doctor-friend told us that we would have to spend two weeks in the hospital. It would take two weeks for the doctors to regulate Danai's diabetes and for us to attend nutritional seminars and courses on how to administer the right amount of insulin to correspond with the amount of nutrition she consumed. All of us—Danai, her father, and me— would need that time to learn how to inject insulin. "Diabetes is a way of life" my Greek friend told me, attempting to console me before she left work on the first night after Danai's diagnosis. But back then, nothing could calm me down. I did not know whether to believe her—or how we would integrate the injections and dangers of diabetes into our lives. I could not imagine how we would go on living with such a serious interruption to our daily routine. How could we behave as if diabetes had always been part of our lives? Perhaps the most serious and difficult obstacle I faced during these first moments was denial. I did not want my daughter to learn to live with diabetes. I did not want to accept the truth.

I believed that two weeks was much too long and that I would become claustrophobic in the hospital, which already made me uncomfortable. What would happen to Ioli? How could I tell her we were spending so many days in the hospital, or that I was staying with her sister and not including her? How could I tell her she would have to go to sleep at night without my being there to read her a story, give her a hug, or say goodnight? What about her swimming class? How could I explain that she wouldn't be able to show me how well she could swim on the last day? In just a few hours, all of our plans had been derailed.

There was no alternative solution. The two-week educational program was required for all children diagnosed with type one diabetes. This timeframe was determined by the hospital and no one was granted a reduction. We would spend these two weeks adjusting, as a family, to an emergency situation. This was the first of many new conditions that would force every member of our family to develop new, more flexible ways of thinking in order to manage our growing inner conflicts.

Living with diabetes "will be like brushing her teeth," a Greek relative said.

I knew he was trying to comfort me, but diabetes could not be compared to brushing teeth, unless one had very problematic teeth that caused pain and side effects throughout the body. I could imagine a diabetic child one day accepting the condition as part of her own reality, but I could not imagine that the demands of diabetes would ever become a completely normal and undisruptive part of our routine—at least, not until different treatments had been developed for this condition.

During our first week in the hospital, Danai was not allowed to go out. We had appointments not only with diabetologists, but also with other specialists. Her blood sugar levels were measured between meals throughout the day, every day, and at regular intervals throughout the entire night, every night. These measurements indicated the amount of insulin she needed at various times of day and night. In the hospital, Danai quickly accepted her diagnosis, and seemed to adjust to the demands of diabetes worryingly fast. She followed the specialists' instructions without any objections. She stood in the kitchen while her food was weighed and learned how to calculate how much of it she could consume, in relation to the amount of insulin she was taking before meals. She started injecting herself with insulin early on and read all of the information the hospital gave us on life as a diabetic. She spent time with the friends who visited her, and they shared news from school. She drew, waited, and listened and was always ready on time for the special classes provided by the hospital. She said, "yes," to everything she was asked to do. She seemed to accept hospital life as an unavoidable part of her routine. The mature behavior of this eight-year-old girl impressed doctors and nurses alike, as well as everyone else who came into contact with her. Danai was certainly a nice surprise and an easy patient for all of the staff on the diabetes ward.

I did not do so well. The day after Danai's diagnosis, I had my first meeting with her doctors in the so-called "parents' room," which was located on the same floor as her own room. After putting up a "please do not disturb" sign and closing the door, the doctors told my husband and me that Danai's lack of symptoms indicated that her diabetes was still at the first stage, which was a good thing. It was good that she had been diagnosed in time, before she developed the aggravating symptoms of hyperglycemia. Although the doctors were trying to reassure us that Danai's diabetes was not very advanced and that she was lucky not to have already fallen into a coma, I found their revelation the most repulsive, ugly, painful, and threatening sequence of sounds I had heard since the diagnosis. The thought that my child could be exposed to so much danger so suddenly and that she could actually fall into a coma shattered all my efforts to use my remaining energy to focus on communicating with the people around me.

"Danai in…" I did not want to complete the thought, although I did want to understand what we had escaped.

"Things have changed" the doctors started telling us, to move the discussion on to something more positive. Diabetics have a much easier time today than in the past, thanks to technological advances. In earlier times, no one survived diabetes because no insulin was available. Another horrific fact: in the past, diabetes was a terminal illness. My imagination was filled with horrible images; the doctors' efforts to encourage me were having the opposite effect. I know now how useful it can be to learn about medical achievements and technological advances in the treatment of diabetes. However, it was much too soon for me to feel grateful for or consoled by the treatments, new inventions, and accomplishments of science. Earlier in my life or during a general discussion of diabetes, I probably would have been more receptive, even admiring the accomplishments of medical specialists. At that particular moment, the diagnosis concerned my own child and I was completely aware of its seriousness. The whole situation took a toll, and I felt I was collapsing physically as well as mentally. There were too many changes taking place too fast. The new reality was extremely demanding and difficult to bear. I did not want to think about how Danai's newly diagnosed condition would affect her—a condition that was permanent and incurable. I did not want to believe that there was no way back. I burst into tears and had difficulties breathing. I watched the doctors' faces as they looked at and talked to me, but I could not communicate or take in what they were saying.

Amid this confusion, Dr. P. called the mobile phone number I had given him, appearing in our midst like a deus ex machina. I left the room to talk to him. It was good to escape from the parents' room and listen to the familiar, soothing voice of Danai's pediatrician. This phone call felt liberating—even life-saving. He had known both of my children since birth, and was someone I trusted, someone who had helped every time they were sick.

Doctor P. wanted to know how far along we were with Danai's diagnosis. I told him that Danai had been diagnosed with type one diabetes and my first question to him was whether or not she could get pregnant. He replied in a reassuring way, even smiling, that yes, she could. This gave me some relief but I could not feel joy. I heard him telling me that I was not alone in this situation, and that I could turn to him or to any other specialist for whatever help I needed. Then our Greek doctor-friend showed up and took me back into the room of oppressive discussions. The information session had to go on. Diabetes was threatening Danai and I could not protect her. I continued to be unable to communicate. As a result, the session had to be postponed to another day.

I knew that whatever my own reaction to Danai's diagnosis of diabetes, it was imperative that I put my own feelings, pain, personal worries, and questions to one side and support my daughter. No matter how cooperative she appeared to be, I knew that Danai was under an enormous amount of pressure. I had to be at her side, doing everything I could to reduce her sense of insecurity and fears about the future. Our past had definitely contributed in a positive way towards creating a shared feeling of safety and peace. Our relationship was based on honesty, trust, and love, which we expressed to each other at different moments in our everyday lives. I would always love Danai, but I could not go on being completely honest with her. I allowed myself to pretend to be cheerful. I smiled when I was not happy. I made jokes when I wanted to cry. I walked and raced with her down the hospital corridors when I longed to huddle in a corner and be quiet and alone with my thoughts, fears, disappointment, and distress.

Whenever I faced a particularly demanding situation, I remembered Darwin's observations on how living beings adapted to changes in their environments. His theory of "the survival of the fittest" really helped me. Those who are willing to adapt fast to whatever change takes place around them are the ones who will survive. Creatures who don't adapt will be known to the planet's inhabitants only through books. They become history. I remembered reading about some beautifully colored butterflies in Manchester, England, which turned into an industrial area at the end of the 19th century. Industrial waste turned the landscape grey, and the colorful butterflies lost their colors in order to survive.

I had always claimed to be a Darwinist and now it was time to prove it. I did not want to abandon colors or sounds—we could survive without having to do that. The steps we had to take to adapt to the new reality were of a different nature. We had to confront our own hurricane of emotions and survive, day in, day out. Our reality, with its new facts and the changes they introduced, was moving faster than light. But our bodies and psyches could not instantly adapt to these changes, especially when they were happening so quickly. The majority of humans have not reached a stage of mental development that enables them to deal instantly and easily with big challenges. Even Manchester's butterflies did not change their color overnight.

Danai's shocking diagnosis and my own inability to accept it gave me psychosomatic symptoms, including hearing problems and sleeping disorders. I knew what a staggering set of changes we were all confronting. Nevertheless, I had to keep functioning to meet our basic needs; to accomplish that, I had to go home.

Our home under normal circumstances was a bright, colorful place with radiant energy, warm, cozy, and joyful. This was not just my own impression but also something many guests had told me, young and old. When I opened the door of our house for the first time after Danai's diagnosis, I froze. The place in front of me was not my home. It was not mine at all. It felt strange; nothing seemed familiar. This place had no colors. I could not hear happy children talking, giggling, or fighting over trivial things. I was frightened by the absolute quiet. Normally, I enjoyed quiet, but at this particular moment, it was torture. The emptiness seemed to be talking to me, telling me that everything had changed and that I had better accept it. I could not relax in my refuge as I had before the diagnosis. It had become inhospitable, as if a cold, strong wind were penetrating each room and pushing me out. Where had all the colors gone? Why had everything turned grey all of a sudden?

I glanced into Danai's room but did not have the courage to enter. I felt it was no longer her room. This was where she had slept before she had diabetes, but now...? The smells, her unmade bed, desk, soft toys, clothes, books, and socks lying on the floor, her beloved jump rope—all these things belonged to the era before diabetes. This was where we used to listen to music and play board games, where we planned her parties, danced, and played blind man's bluff. This was where we used to hug and say how much we loved each other. Here Danai and I read bedtime stories and I switched off the light without measuring her blood sugar, without injections or hypoglycemia. How could I let all this go? Why did this reality abandon me so cruelly and heartlessly? Where did we go wrong? What could I have done to prevent this? I couldn't bear this much longer. It was torture. I left everything lying where it was, without touching anything. I turned away—feeling the sorrow of so much loss.

I approached my office. The last time I had used it, I'd known nothing about insulin injections or sugar level measurements. I had not been worried about my child's health or even aware of the existence of the diabetes ward in our local hospital. Taking small steps, in a cowardly way, I approached the papers piled up on my desk. I'd been studying them on Monday, before Danai came back from school and we went to the pediatrician's office. I'd made her appointment from this office that day. Everything here had remained in the pre-diabetes era. The last time I had looked at these papers, I'd had no idea that my daughter's pancreas was not functioning properly. I'd been making notes, believing that life had been generous to me. The only thing I'd had to do was study when my children were away from home, so that I could take my psychology final exams at the university and get my degree. My only real worry had been whether I would do well on those exams, a serious challenge. Although this part of my life was quite recent, it now felt as if centuries lay between this moment and then.

I looked at my papers and notes, but did not dare to turn over a single page. I did not want to touch anything in that room where, under different circumstances, I would have spent many hours of the day and night. I felt that someone else must have lived here and used this office. Someone else had written those notes on all of those texts. Someone else. Not me. I did not want to be in the house anymore, so I took what I needed, dropped off what I no longer needed, and escaped as fast as I could. I could not stand to compare our lives after diabetes with our lives before, as represented by everything I saw in these rooms. It was a relief to get back to the hospital.

I did not want the children to remember our stay in the hospital as a traumatic experience. For that reason, I started adding some variety and interest to our days there. Instead of having the same kind of dinner every evening, with the same bread, cheese, and butter day after day, we would sometimes order pizza from our favorite pizza place. We would then all wait in the outer corridor of the diabetes ward, near the elevators, for the pizza man in his red uniform. We looked forward to seeing him arrive in place of the usual doctors, nurses, sick children in wheelchairs with needles in their arms dispensing medications, pale, silent children lying motionless on their beds, cleaning staff, and healthcare specialists. At these special moments, we waited for the pizza man to show up as a fisherman waits for his catch. When the elevator door opened and revealed him balancing with one hand the insulating bag that kept the pizza warm, we felt almost ecstatic. The smell of the pizza reminded me that life was going on out there without us and that we mustn't forget to live it to the full, once we returned to the outside world.

Some days after we arrived, I also transformed Danai's hospital bed. At the first opportunity, I went to the children's favorite toy store and came back carrying a big, soft, pink horse, small magnetic paper horses, and some other items to turn the place where Danai would have to spend so many days into a child-friendly environment. I entered her room loaded with loot and threw the big pink horse into her arms. Horse riding was Danai's favorite sport and she naturally adored horses. This was the best I could offer her, under the circumstances, to create the illusion that she was close to the animals she loved so much. The soft, pink horse occupied the whole lower half of Danai's bed. On top of the big white hospital pillow, I spread a colorful towel with pictures of running horses, and Danai stuck the little horse magnets on her bed frame, breaking up the monotonous hospital white. If we had to stay so long, I thought, we should at least bring some color into our lives again.

I also made some changes to the décor in our home. The pediatric clinic was bursting with illustrations of different themes, and the walls and glass doors of the diabetes ward were covered with images related to the sea: boats, whales, octopuses, fish, sea stars, and shells. I discovered where I could get the same designs and put them up in our own bathroom at home, so that with each new visit to the hospital, the children would feel (at least unconsciously) a bit more at home. I had the feeling that this would not be our last hospital stay.

As this was going on, we also had meetings with specialists of all sorts. The protocol of the diabetes ward required the parents of diabetic children to learn to how to administer injections, so that they could inject their children with insulin whenever necessary. The next expert to attempt to train us was Mrs. H., who should have been called, "Mrs. In-a-Hurry," a special counselor for families with diabetic children. Her manner was superficially cheerful and charming, but also arrogant and stress-inducing. She told my husband and me to come to her office the next day to attend her class. We were led to understand that this very important but extremely busy hospital staff member was unfortunately always under enormous time pressure. She emphasized that we should be careful not to be late and made us feel that she was doing us a favor by devoting time to us.

The next day, we showed up promptly at Mrs. In-a-Hurry's office and then waited for a considerable amount of time for her to be ready to receive us. It was a tiny room full of brochures on diabetes, syringes, insulin tubes, and gifts for small children (such as soft toys) from pharmaceutical companies, all squeezed onto very few shelves, and piled up on every surface. It also had no window, which added to my discomfort. Mrs. In-a-Hurry started the meeting by bragging about her irreplaceable contribution to the functioning of the hospital's diabetes ward. She let us know that she was considering many job offers, some from distant countries, because she was unhappy with her employers, who did not allow her to serve families in the way she considered right.

While Mrs. In-a-Hurry was narcissistically engaged, I noticed a little card lying on the table; on it was written: "the owner of this card is diabetic." A blank space was provided in the margin so that parents could add their telephone number and that of the diabetic child's doctor. In addition, the card explained to whoever found it what to do if the child was in a coma. Feeling shattered, I started shivering. What sort of world did we live in now? What would my child's life be like from now on? Would she constantly face such great danger that she would need to carry this card with her at all times? The message implied that strangers would have to help her immediately. What if something like this happened and I wasn't there? Who would help her? How would they help her? What kind of life would Danai lead from now on? I suddenly felt an unbearable pain.

For Mrs. In-a-Hurry, who had been advising the families of diabetic children for who knows how long, all of this information was taken for granted. She didn't even bother to explain the little diabetic's card lying on the table. It was just part of her routine and the way she ran her office; she wanted it to be right where she had placed it. She did not have the slightest inkling how shocking this little piece of text could be to the mother of a newly diagnosed diabetic child. Of course, the purpose of this card was to help diabetic children facing dangerous situations. The fact was that Danai had been diagnosed with diabetes and here was another icy professional doing her job in the most insensitive way possible. Although I was shaken, I had to accept our new situation there and then.

I had to live up to the demands of the moment. Our assignment for the day was to learn from this special advisor how to inject insulin. We had to learn from scratch how to prepare an injection, which type of insulin went into the syringe first, and which second, where the bubbles were supposed to go, which way the needle had to go in, how fast to force insulin out of the plastic tube and under the skin, how long to wait before removing the needle from the diabetic's body, and how quickly to give injections. Our schedule required us to pierce our own thighs and bellies in order to feel what it was like to insert a needle into the body and remove it at the right speed. It was important to have a good command of all this information for Danai's sake.

For her sake, I was willing to be patient and put up with everything I was asked to perform. But Mrs. In-a-Hurry managed one more slap in the face, hurting me with a stunningly inconsiderate comment, made while demonstrating the skills we needed to learn. "Just think," she said, in her arrogant way, "when Danai is at a disco, she will have to go into the bathroom and squeeze her arm against the wall like junkies do, in order to be able to inject insulin with her other hand." There was no good reason to make us imagine this scene, not only because Danai was only eight years old and could not possibly go to a disco, but also because it was horrible to think of our daughter needing to hide in a public bathroom to give herself an insulin injection. The picture that Mrs. In-a-Hurry forced us to imagine was devastating, making me worry uncontrollably about Danai's future.

How much of this could I put up with? I started to cry, realizing how serious our situation really was. I thought about my child, and how she would always be dependent on injections. I cried because there was nothing I could do to change this reality. I cried because my daughter would not be able to take a bus or walk down the street on her own until she was sixteen. The general fear of hypoglycemia was unmistakable. Our meeting ended then and Mrs. In-a-Hurry's arrogant and austere instruction (was there even a hint of sadism?) was temporarily interrupted. We arranged to meet and continue our training on another morning.

The ordeal went on and on. Every Wednesday morning, a Professor of Diabetics who was a distinguished expert visited the ward to meet diabetic children and their parents and ask them all sorts of questions. This was a meeting I would not miss, no matter where I was or what I was doing. So on Wednesday morning I stayed next to Danai, who was lying in bed, and waited for his visit. I wanted to meet him and hear what he had to say. Our Greek doctor-friend had told me that parents and their diabetic children would travel long distances to hear his views. He entered the room escorted by a large group of medical staff members from other departments, all dressed in white. There were trainee doctors and other diabetologists, as well as Mrs. D., the nutrition expert, and the pediatric clinic's psychiatrist—all standing quietly and waiting for him to speak.

The Professor of Diabetics was the only person who asked questions. He asked Danai how everything was going. How was she supposed to reply to him or describe her feelings when, just a few hours earlier, she had learned that she would have to inject herself for the rest of her life? Danai gave him a dejected look. The doctor, who was trying in his own way to establish a friendly relationship, told her that diabetic children were good at mathematics because they were always having to calculate the right amount of food to match the insulin they had to take. Five years have passed since that moment, but I am absolutely certain that he was the only one who smiled. I could not see any amusement on Danai´s face. I only remember her looking at him—helpless, speechless, and sad.

Then it was my turn. He wanted to know whether I had started injecting my child. "No" was the answer. He did not like that. I had to do it, he said, without thinking for a moment what he was asking me to do. To this doctor—a Professor of Diabetics—it seemed absolutely natural that I should be ready and able to stick a needle into my daughter´s body, although I hadn't graduated from medical school or any similar program. He ordered me to begin injecting my child, an act which felt synonymous with pain and injury. Only days after Danai´s admission to the hospital, this gentleman expected me to put my feelings aside and pierce my daughter's body; he made me feel as if I had committed a crime by not having done it yet. He stared at me fixedly, his blue eyes like two imaginary stabbing needles. Of course, I had to do it! I should be able, as a mother, to inject my child, he lectured me, in front of the large group of white-clad observers. Although I told him that I understood my duties, the conversation made me feel really uncomfortable. It felt as if he were assuming I could fly an airplane just because I could drive a car.

The next question he asked, in front of Danai, was whether anyone else in the family had diabetes. There was one relative: my father. What, how, when, how much—the Professor asked every personal question he could think of. It did not cross his mind that he might be upsetting my child or me. Children's souls were sacrificed on the altar of research that morning. When the doctor wanted to know whether I had any questions, I asked whether we could continue our discussion in private another time, without Danai present and the eyes of so many specialists appraising us.

Fortunately, the doctor agreed. He was not unkind; he just lacked the fine intuition that a doctor needs to work with distressed people. He did not know how far to push his demands or when to stop challenging a wounded person. The next day, I had a private meeting with this doctor and asked him twenty questions about diabetes and Danai's future. We were able to have a friendly and relaxed discussion. He reassured me that, if we did not feel ready to leave the hospital after two weeks, he would not send us home. We could stay in the hospital until we felt safe going out into the world. However, the scheduled Wednesday morning visit left scars, as I had been afraid it would.

"I can thank your father for this," Danai said, guessing that she had probably inherited her diabetes from my father. Who was the mediator of this inheritance? Me, of course. Feelings of guilt began to overwhelm me. Why had Danai inherited diabetes when I carry the gene and don't have it? Did this happen because I shouted at her when she blew out the candles on her sister's birthday cake a month before the diagnosis? What could have I done differently to avoid this situation? Wasn't I a good enough mother?

I started asking why Danai had contracted diabetes. The only thing that was certain was that no one could tell me with any certainty what conditions caused diabetes to manifest in children. According to statistical data, more cases are diagnosed in the Scandinavian countries. Since there isn't much sun in that part of the world, some suspect that a lack of sunshine could be a possible trigger for type one diabetes. The condition also occurs in children whose relatives are diabetes-free. Something as simple as a cold, the doctors told me, could cause part of the pancreas to malfunction. The organism mistakenly turns against itself and destroys parts of the organ responsible for the production of insulin. Some months before Danai was diagnosed, we had spent our Christmas vacation in Athens. She had written to Santa in "his" hut in downtown Athens: "I want to get rid of my cold. Happy New Year. Danai!" Did that cold cause everything that was to follow some months later? How many colds do people catch in a lifetime and how many times do they avoid contracting type one diabetes? Why would Danai´s body make such a serious mistake? What was the reason for all this happening?

5. UNSOLICITED VISITORS

Danai's recently diagnosed diabetes was not the only situation causing us discomfort. We also had to cope with waves of uninvited visitors—people (both friends and acquaintances) whose comments only increased my worries and insecurities. Just a few days after Danai's admission to the hospital, the diabetes ward was swarming with people who apparently believed that the best way to improve my morale was to bother me with mindless comments and opinions.

Many of them seemed to have come as a purely automatic response, or simply out of curiosity, perhaps reflecting the way they were socialized in childhood. These people must have learned early on that fulfilling social obligations, such as visiting the sick and their families in hospitals, was a wise and decent thing to do. They made a show of being friendly, but did not want to invest any real time or emotion. They had no interest in offering practical help. In our case, for example, it would have been wonderful if one of the many passers-by had offered to entertain little loli for a few hours while her family was in the hospital, struggling to familiarize itself with the unknown and demanding world of diabetes. No one who visited ever made such an offer. I wished that most of our visitors would just stay home or go anywhere else, rather than coming to the hospital to overload me with their views and knowledge on diabetes.

"It must be related to some sort of traumatic event your child experienced in the family" a "friend" told me, without seeming to consider the impact of her words or the damage she was causing. This woman knew of another child who had developed diabetes after his parents got divorced.

I felt this comment as a blow. My inner world began to shake. I felt naked and exposed out there in the cold, egocentric adult world. My initial reaction was to try to think of a traumatic event that could have caused Danai to develop this condition. Was it perhaps when she hurt her face falling off a skateboard on her way home from school? Was this injury such a shock that it disrupted her body? Before I could draw any conclusions or put myself under further psychological strain, I realized that if traumatic experiences caused type one diabetes, more than half the world's people would be carrying insulin in their pockets.

The next authority on diabetes was the mother of one of Danai's friends. She wanted to protect us from the dangers of diabetes and hypoglycemia, especially during the night. Her sources had informed her that diabetics with low blood sugar levels could get up in the middle of the night and walk through glass doors. She just wanted us to know that. This sort of insensitive attitude made me even more physically and mentally exhausted.

Five years later, I cannot forget the desperation, insecurity, and pain caused by these and other similar comments. I will never forget the emptiness in my heart when I thought about the future. Such personal encounters made me cautious in the presence of anyone with a professed interest in diabetes. So many people expressed insincere interest, compassion, and understanding. It was particularly hard for me to deal with those who combined an expression of sorrow with obvious indifference. Such behavior seems to me a cheap and dishonest way of reducing humanity to a state of wretchedness, especially those experiencing hardships. These hospital encounters made me suspect that those who treat people in difficult situations this way are indirectly expressing a sense of triumph: how lucky they are to be better off than the sufferer or victim standing before them! What's worse is that this behavior can be expressed in the cheapest, most humiliating and cunning ways imaginable. The visitor or spectator appears to make a quick comparison, assessing his or her own position in relation to that of the sufferer, before exuding a sense of superiority.

During our stay in the hospital, I became aware of the fact that many people visit patients and their families in order to verify through direct contact (most of the time, I believe, unconsciously) how lucky they are to enjoy a better destiny. They are basically reassuring themselves that they are the children of a kinder God. They leave the patients and families they have visited feeling proud, relieved, and satisfied with themselves, with no inkling of how much damage they have caused through their inappropriate, clumsy comments. Such people return to their petty, selfish, and presumably monotonous routines, patting themselves on the backs for the successful fake lives they have managed to create.

Danai's school teacher was such a person. I was surprised when she expressed an interest in coming to visit, as she had not up to then seemed to love her job or be particularly interested in or fond of children. She was certainly not someone who generally engaged in loving acts. Even as a very young child, Danai had always had excellent instincts, carefully observing and assessing other people. This woman had been her teacher for three years, and I knew from Danai's daily comments that she had never been a real advisor, loving guide, or affectionate companion in learning.

Despite all this, we could not prevent her from visiting. Perhaps we wanted to give her a chance to prove that we had underestimated her. So the teacher came to the hospital one evening after work. She took a chair and sat next to Danai's bed, while I stood nearby, observing her. My naiveté made me expect her to express some tenderness or compassion for the odyssey this eight-year-old child was going through. I thought she might even be amusing. But the connection between child and teacher was cold and uncomfortable. I could understand how Danai felt—this visitor was her teacher, not a friend with whom she could talk freely. The teacher was silent and emotionless, and I wondered why she had wanted to visit. She stared hard at Danai, making her feel awkward. Her silence was catching; Danai did not utter a word.

I decided to break the ice with a comment about the big pink horse that was spread out across the whole bed.

"Every child who has visited Danai would love to have this horse, but only Danai can have it," I said. I froze as I heard the teacher say: "Yeah, but no child wants to have your disease, Danai!"

Danai just nodded at this unexpected blow. She did not have the power to defend herself, and felt abashed at this comment from her teacher, a woman paid to mess with human souls. I wanted to confront her myself, but did not want to make things difficult for my child, who would have to return to this teacher's class when she went back to school.

I had to meet this teacher outside class some days later, to give her a document from the hospital. I talked to her about how to treat Danai when she returned to school. My daughter should not be pitied, I said. "You don't need to feel sorry for her." She looked puzzled. "No?" she marveled. "No," I reassured her. I could tell that she did not understand the importance of what I was asking her to do. I gave up trying to educate this educator. The voices of children in Danai's classroom upset me and I felt my daughter's absence acutely. She was in the hospital facing huge challenges. Just a few days ago, she had been playing and laughing in school, with no suspicion of what was to follow. I could not bear the enormous contrast between those two situations; I could not bear to hear the voices of her classmates, laughing and playing innocently, while my child was already losing this innocence and learning to live with injections and hypoglycemia. I left the school and returned to her as fast as I could.

6. THE OPPRESSIVE MEETINGS CONTINUE

Many times, I have wondered which is more catastrophic for the diabetic person and his or her family: diabetes itself or the maliciousness and ignorance of people who move within a bubble of selfish behavior. I suspect that the harm human beings inflict through inappropriate behavior, as a result of terrifying selfishness, is much greater than the problems caused by diabetes.

We have been fortunate, however, to be surrounded not only by people in bubbles, but also by advanced minds who genuinely want to help others and to sooth their sorrow and pain. I met someone like this at the hospital. He accompanied the nutrition advisor, whose job it was to teach us how to calculate the number of carbohydrates consumed during main meals and snacks. To train us, the nutrition expert showed up at one of our morning meetings pushing a supermarket trolley filled with all sorts of unknown products: empty bottles of various soft drinks, different sorts of junk food wrappers, plastic sausages and other sorts of meat, plastic bread rolls, and fast food—all samples of our "daily nutrition." It was not the healthiest menu in the world, but I guess it was supposed to represent the eating habits of the majority of people in Europe.

My problem was not the unhealthy products in the shopping cart. I was confident that I could figure out how to calculate the carbohydrates in the sort of food we normally ate at home. My problem was that, once again—in a very short period of time—I was confronted by all the enormous changes that we, and especially Danai, were facing. Comparing our lives before and after upset me so much that my eyes filled with tears and I could not follow what the nutritionist was saying. I could not calculate how many carbohydrates were in the piece of food she was showing me. I could not even see her face clearly. This expert rushed through the process and our first attempt to learn about nutritional issues ended sooner than scheduled.

Alarmed by this incident, the nutritionist contacted the department's child psychiatrist. He specialized in the problems faced by families beginning to live with diabetes. A day after my meeting with the nutritionist, she and the psychiatrist found me at the end of the diabetes ward corridor, where there were board games piled onto a few shelves and some children's chairs and tables. I was playing a game with Danai. We sat next to the window and glanced outside between throws of the dice. From that vantage point, I could watch people passing by. I guessed that most of them had no idea what it meant to be type one diabetic.

Before the psychiatrist could introduce himself, I approached him and told him that I knew who he was. I took him to one side to arrange a meeting with the whole family, as he had suggested. I wanted to talk to Danai personally about this counselor. The meeting took place shortly after that, perhaps even a day later, in his office on the fourth floor of the hospital, with a psychologist also present. Both the psychiatrist and the psychologist wanted to know how we all felt now that diabetes was part of our lives. The children seemed lost in this new and unknown situation; they were too young to feel comfortable describing how they felt, especially to a stranger. I therefore suggested to both experts that it would be better to talk without the children present.

We let the two girls go back to the diabetes ward. There was no reason to trouble two young children and force them describe what was obvious. The psychologist took advantage of the children's departure to ask me how I felt about having to give Danai injections. Apparently, he had been told by diabetes ward staff members that I was still unable to face the excruciating ordeal of piercing my child's body with a needle, despite having been told a number of times that I must. I did not answer. There was so much I could have said, all obvious, all depressing. The psychologist undertook the task of analyzing my inner world. I had no objection to that. I was afraid, he supposed, that I would injure Danai's body. Yes, that was true. I also had to overcome many other obstacles in order to feel able to inject insulin into my daughter. One key obstacle was an inability to accept the new reality.

For our next appointment, I met the psychiatrist alone, without my husband, who seemed to have accepted the new situation stoically. The psychiatrist wanted to hear about my feelings that particular morning. The night before, I had slept at home, as it was Ioli's turn to have her Mom. Back then, I'd felt completely overwhelmed and this had affected my physical condition as well as my sleeping routine. That morning, as I lay in bed, I was thinking of the unexpected turn Danai's life had taken, and how this was also affecting other members of the family. I described my psychological condition to the psychiatrist through a vision, something like a waking dream that I'd had while resting but alert. This vision revealed my psychological state hours after the diagnosis. I described it to help this kind-hearted man understand how I was feeling—not just that morning, but in general:

"That morning," I told him, "I saw myself standing in a Greek island port watching a ship depart. The port was deserted, and I was the only figure there. I could feel sorrow spreading inside me as I watched the bright, vivid lights of the ship. I could hear music and the voices of people enjoying themselves. I thought that this was my life before the diagnosis of diabetes, a life now deserting me. Where I was standing in the colorless, lifeless, cold port, without movement, people, voices, or music—that was my life now. The life unfolding ahead of me was silent, cold, and colorless, without the affection or warmth I used to take for granted."

I remember the psychiatrist remaining silent for some seconds. I could see the effort he was making not to reveal how much my words had affected him. What could he say to make me feel better? Nothing at all, and that was all I wanted to hear. All I wanted was for him to understand how weighed down I felt by my daughter's recent diagnosis. I hoped he would know how the mother of a child newly diagnosed with diabetes must feel, without my having to explain. The psychiatrist wanted to know how I was feeling and I gave him an honest answer. I even told him a thought that had crossed my mind: if I didn't have children, I wouldn't have to go through so much pain. This thought was immediately followed by a second, that I could not imagine my life without this child, without Danai, no matter how much pain I was feeling.

When you truly love, you love without conditions or special agreements. When you become a parent, you do not sign a contract with your fate, agreeing to play the role only as long as the scenario remains a comedy. That is not pure love or real giving. When I decided to become a mother, I took a conscious decision. After this meeting, the psychiatrist working with the families of diabetic children never asked to see me again. He just greeted me in his own sweet, humane way every time we accidentally met in the hospital.

As the days passed by, we followed the hospital's schedule for families new to the world of type one diabetes. At our next appointment with Mrs. In-a-Hurry, my husband and I found ourselves back in her tiny office. We were there to learn to deal with insulin injections, as time was passing and all the "musts" encroaching. Mrs. In-a-Hurry's egocentricity and narcissism remained an obstacle, but there was no alternative to this training session. Like it or not, we had to work with this woman as best we could.

She informed us that she had pierced her body with a syringe a number of times, as part of her job. However, she could not afford to do this every time she came into contact with beginners (new parents learning how to inject their children). Pharmaceutical companies had come up with a solution to that problem and provided dummies, small cushions covered with advertisements for medical equipment. Using these cushions, the counselor showed us how to inject our own bodies.

Now it was our turn. First in line was my husband. He had to inject his belly and get used to the feeling of doing it. Without hesitation, he followed the protocol and thrust the needle into his belly, while pressing down with the fingers of his other hand to make the skin curve before the needle entered his body. Then, following the instructions of the expert, who was now observing every single movement he made, he removed the needle from his body at the right speed, so as to avoid injury or pain.

Very pleased with the performance of Danai's very composed and cooperative father, Mrs. In-a-Hurry reassured him that he was now qualified to inject his daughter. He accepted her assessment. In this restricted space, I remember the figure of a trainee doctor sitting opposite us and silently observing the whole procedure, as part of her own training. She had asked our permission to observe us while we experimented with needles and tubes, and we had agreed.

I was next in line. The moment I never wanted to come had arrived. I felt that I was being forced violently inside some kind of pressing machine—any minute someone outside would press a button and start squeezing my soul. The feeling materialized—Mrs. In-a-Hurry pressed the squeezing button. She asked me to inject my belly. My belly? Why on earth my belly? What about all the other parts of my body? I refused. My belly was my child's first home—the same child who was now waiting in her bed in the diabetes ward for me to learn to inject her body.

Memories of being pregnant with Danai flooded my mind at lightning speed. I felt the indescribable joy of pregnancy and the indescribable sorrow of Danai's diagnosis colliding at high speed and tearing me to pieces. I did not want to use this part of my body to learn to give insulin injections. I did not want any needle for any reason to penetrate my child's first home.

Inside this home, Danai had grown in an environment of love. I was sure that she had felt loved, judging from how she had developed before and after birth. Now, some years later, I could not shield her from psychological and physical pain; her life depended on insulin injections. These rapid comparisons aroused intense, real feelings that overwhelmed me. Sobs shook my whole body. My husband suggested to the counselor that it would be better if he and the trainee doctor left the room, so that I would not feel the pressure of being observed under such demanding conditions.

The request was granted. I remained alone with the trainer to do what had to be done. There was an alternative: to try to inject my thigh. I grabbed the opportunity. I followed the expert's instructions and injected myself correctly. The needle was really tiny and hardly noticeable. I did not feel any pain. That was good. Danai would not feel pain, I hoped. It was good to try to experience for a moment what my child would experience from then on, in her now unpredictable future. Now I was qualified to do the same thing with my daughter's thigh, Mrs. In-a-Hurry pronounced. I knew I wasn't ready for such a performance and wouldn't be ready for a long time, even when I was actually giving Danai injections. Even the suggestion felt threatening. However, Mrs. In-a-Hurry didn't allow thoughts or feelings to interfere with deeds. In any case, she was in a hurry to get to her next appointment. She told me that on the next day, I would have to give Danai her morning injection in the presence of nurses.

I was honest and confessed that I wouldn't feel safe in that situation. I had the impression that some of the nurses were not highly qualified and did not know enough about diabetes. I would not feel secure while making my first attempt to give Danai an injection. I was not sure that any nurse would be able to give me the right sort of help if I needed It. Mrs. In-a-Hurry surprised me with a special offer: she was willing to meet me in Danai's room the next morning, without the nurses, to supervise my first insulin injection. This was a good solution and a good compromise; it made me hope that I could manage to accomplish this task, which had felt impossible before.

Time passed at the hospital; the nurses measured Danai's blood sugar levels, supervised insulin injections, weighed food, and readjusted the amount of insulin, while doctors paid visits. I spent this time worrying about whether I would be able to cope with so many demands and handle an enormous responsibility: to protect Danai from the possible complications of diabetes. I knew I had no choice. I had to force myself to give her an insulin injection for her own sake. I had to learn to cope with this because, as our Greek doctor-friend had told me, there would be times when Danai might not be willing or able to inject herself with insulin, either because she was tired or for some other reason. I had to be in a position to help. I wanted to help, not just then, but always. I wanted to bring up my daughter in a positive way, but I never could have imagined what my duties as a mother would involve.

As agreed, Mrs. In-a-Hurry and I met the next morning in Danai's room, to give the injection. I knew how to prepare the syringe by mixing together two different sorts of insulin. I had paid careful attention to Mrs. In-a-Hurry's class the day before and remembered the necessary steps in the right order. It was the procedure I had followed when injecting myself. But now, in Danai's room, it felt like the final countdown. I had to start the procedure immediately. As I began, my hands handled the equipment competently and my memory was clear. My performance was flawless at the start. I successfully mixed different amounts of the two different sorts of insulin, impressing Mrs. In-a-Hurry so much that she forgot herself and praised me.

However, this wasn't the hard part; I still had to give Danai an injection in her thigh for the first time. It was a difficult moment, one of many I had recently faced. I looked at my child's leg and my heart ached, even before I tried to give the injection. I remembered that her pediatrician had confessed to me some years earlier that he could not vaccinate his own children and had to ask a colleague to do it. But I was not a doctor and could not engage someone else to give multiple injections to Danai on a daily basis, wherever she was, relieving me of this difficult responsibility.

The counselor reminded me not to think too much about it, but to do what I had to do quickly, because she was very busy and had to leave soon. This was a very important moment for me, and it felt incongruous to have this woman standing next to me, bragging about how busy she was and hurrying me along. To her, this experience was just part of her own job. My daughter's leg was not her daughter's leg. My daughter's psyche was not her daughter's psyche. For years, she had been giving orders to young and old, in return for which her bank account had received a quantity of cash every month.

I gave Danai the injection as this woman with thick curly hair instructed me to. Her hair looked thicker and curlier every time she sliced through the hospital corridors in her supercilious, arrogant, authoritarian way. When she walked, her whole body moved up and down in an exaggerated manner. She almost jumped from foot to foot in her high heels, while at the same time trying to balance on them, making herself as noticeable as possible to anyone lucky enough to be nearby. Her hair and the face it framed seemed somehow fake and unnatural. A fake person can't understand authentic feelings. She did not understand that this experience would be imprinted on my memory forever. Because she was not genuinely empathetic, she could not guess that five years later, even after giving Danai hundreds of injections, I would always feel a lump in my throat when I thought about the first time.

"Does it hurt, Danai?" I asked her, the moment the miniature needle entered her thigh—a foreign body inside a beloved body. Before my child could answer, the expert spoke for her.

"Ponas? Ponas?" (Does it hurt?) She repeated the Greek word in a bad accent, like a parrot. It was one of the few Greek words she had picked up. "No, it doesn't hurt," Mrs. In-a-Hurry immediately responded with an air of triumph. According to her, this was the right answer. She wasn't interested in giving us a chance to speak or even think.

Perhaps this woman wanted to help in her own way. I could not share her pleasure and satisfaction at having finally convinced me to give Danai an injection. Although we were together in that room, our roles were so different that they could not be compared.

7. SHORT EXPERIMENTS— SHORT ESCAPES

Out of the hospital but only for a few minutes...

After spending several days in the hospital, we were allowed to take Danai away from the diabetes ward. At first, it was only for a limited period of time, within the hospital grounds. We were grateful for this freedom. It was Fall but the weather was still pleasant and we very much wanted to get out and enjoy the fresh air, so different from the hospital atmosphere. We wanted to have a walk and try to forget what had happened only hours before. We wanted to feel as if we still existed.

Danai was permitted to use the elevator only under adult supervision, and never without essential first aid equipment for hypoglycemia, even if she was only leaving the building for four or five minutes. We took everything we needed: the device for measuring blood sugar and some juice and cookies—and then we left. Outside, Danai was running and jumping, feeling happy about her first escape from the diabetes ward. I understood her uplifted spirits without being able to share them. I still felt that my body was wounded and my soul battered, but for my child's sake, I had to force both to function as well as possible.

What had happened was good, I thought. I would carry this load on my own shoulders because I wanted Danai to be able to live as much as possible as a child. We stamped on the dry autumn leaves, which had come to the end of their circle of life and left the tree that had created them. This was something we loved to do at this time of the year, saying to each other that when you stamp on dry leaves it sounds like crunching potato chips. Everything moves in a circle, I thought. Life comes and goes. Trampling dry leaves this time was completely different from the last time.

On our first escape from the hospital, the knowledge that my child was diabetic gave everything a different color. I had to create a new world from scratch, with new rules and new dimensions. I was consciously trying to dismiss the fear and insecurity that threatened me, in order to make Danai believe that she wasn't in any danger and could run and chase leaves without worrying about hypoglycemia. I felt that if we weren't brave from the start, if we didn't dare to live under this constant threat, diabetes would defeat us.

Only days after Danai´s admission to the hospital, we had managed to settle into our room. In this room, we had our meals and studied hospital brochures and books about diabetes. In this room, we showered and slept—Danai in her bed and me beside her on a folding divan. Everything was scheduled: when the room was cleaned, when teams of doctors would visit with questions, and when we would eat breakfast, lunch, and dinner. The measuring of Danai's blood sugar levels and the calculation of her insulin dosage continued until the doctors could estimate how much insulin she needed every hour of the day and night, in order to meet her body´s needs. Discussion after discussion, information, questions, and answers were our daily routine. In just a few days, we had become very familiar with the once strange hospital environment and the previously unknown building and white-clad staff, who were now taking care of Danai. Luckily, as time passed, the acquaintances who visited mainly to satisfy their own curiosity stopped coming and we were left with closer friends, people I could confide in and ask for advice.

Going to town

 As soon as we had completed more advanced training, we were allowed to leave the hospital for a few hours and go further away. The doctors wanted us to pay a short visit to the shops to test our ability to manage the demands of Danai's diabetes under natural living conditions, without the supervision of specialized personnel. It was our first attempt to venture out into the real world and learn to live without the fear that we could not survive outside the hospital. It was also a good opportunity to buy something that would become Danai's permanent companion on every sort of outing: a small pouch to hold essentials needed for living with diabetes.

So the four of us visited various shops and felt that we were on an important mission. That very first family jaunt outside the hospital made me feel once again how much had changed during the past few days. Although the buildings and streets were just as they had been before the diagnosis, nothing seemed the same. I had never before been so anxious about Danai's safety as I was now, watching her walk through store aisles with loli, exploring and picking up items, far away from the noise of the hospital machines, the constant measuring of her blood sugar levels, and the doctors and nurses telling her how to live. She seemed to have already forgotten everything that had happened a few hours before.

On our first trip outside the hospital, I felt anxious and tight, bathed in tension and fear. I could feel only the rhythms of diabetes; nothing else around me mattered. I did not know whether Danai's body was close to hypoglycemia, or whether this short excursion to the shops would be enough to cause some sort of complication. I knew that my husband was also worrying; both of us were on the alert, with nerves stretched tight like thick ropes. Of course, we did not want to show her how we felt. We believed that Danai had the right to be lost in the familiar and beloved world of toys. She had the right to feel her old childlike insouciance. We just had to wait until it was time to measure her blood sugar levels and not panic or remind her of the condition prematurely.

I felt relieved when, for this purpose, we found a drug store, as it was similar to the hospital. At last we could check on her without making her feel that we were worried. The pharmacist showed empathy and a willingness to help. We went behind a folding screen so that Danai could measure her blood sugar levels. It comforted us to find understanding and an offer of practical help. We then had to estimate, without weighing her food or consulting an experienced diabetes nurse, how many carbohydrates Danai could consume. Everything we did during this outing, we did for the first time. Compared to the way we used to be in the pre-diabetes era, every step we took was time-consuming and an effort.

Leaving the hospital for the first time was a real challenge and I was relieved when it was time to go back. I felt safe in there; I did not need to test myself in the outside world. This was where I wanted to be: close to trained staff who knew exactly what it meant to be diabetic. The non-diabetic world was just a burden. I did not want to have to explain our situation. I did not want to hear my neighbor say, "Luckily, my daughters have nothing to do with this horrible disease." I did not want to have to hear people's comments and see their reactions, most of which just satisfied their own egos. I did not want to watch people pretending to be sad about the situation we were in. I did not need anyone's pity. I could manage very well without people's petty "contributions" to my efforts to survive. After getting through the first terrifying crisis of the diagnosis, Danai seemed to adjust to living in the hospital, without realizing what this all meant for her future. She lived only in the present, perhaps because she was so young or perhaps as a defense mechanism— her way of bearing this burden. I did not instigate any discussions about how she felt about having diabetes. We played games, read books, and laughed with the volunteer doctors dressed as clowns who were working hard to amuse the children and their guardians. These relaxing moments were an escape from the reality that lay heavy upon us.

8. THE NEXT EXPERIMENT—THE FIRST VISIT HOME

After our small jaunt to the shops, it was time for a short visit home. There, we would have to weigh Danai's food, inject her insulin, have lunch, and then return to the hospital. Never before had going home for lunch felt like an act of punishment—risky and unwelcome. How would we survive without specialized personnel? I remembered bringing the newborn Danai home from the clinic for the first time. Back then, my worries and fears were very different from the ones I faced now. I worried that I would not be able to change my baby's diaper without the midwife to help me. I was afraid I would not manage to breastfeed her without an advisor permanently beside me. Now the flow of events demanded that we move on to a new stage of evolution in our life with diabetes. We had to abandon the safety of the hospital and test ourselves under natural living conditions.

I remember our whole family sitting around the veranda table, eating. I don't remember what we were eating. Perhaps noodles, the children's favorite dish after stuffed vegetables. I will never forget how numb we all felt. That moment is imprinted in my memory like a film in slow motion, as if gravity had ceased to have an effect on us. I could not avoid the terrifying, disastrous, automatic comparison of our lives before and after the diabetes era. We were having lunch at home for the first time with diabetes among us, at the same table. We were using the chairs we had used before Danai's diagnosis. Over and over, I experienced the same psychological paradox. Although everything around us had remained the same, in some more fundamental way, everything had changed. I am sure I wasn't the only one to feel this—why else did we all behave like wounded animals? Why were we all eating in silence, thinking and worrying?

I tried to pretend that everything was under control, that everything was manageable. We could carry on living in this house just like before. But I knew I was just covering up fresh wounds. I felt that our souls were balancing on a very thin string, that some crisis was about to threaten each one of us. The new crisis did not take long to manifest. We were no ordinary family eating lunch in a familiar environment; after the strange period of silence, Danai finally spoke. She looked sad, very different from the way she had been at the hospital. In a tremulous voice, the eight-year-old girl asked a serious question, expressing the insecurity she felt about her future:

"Am I going to be injecting myself all my life?" she asked, with tears trickling down her cheeks. Then she desperately waited for an answer.

I'm sure this was one of the few moments in Danai's life when she couldn't enjoy the food she was eating, merely swallowing in order to survive. A few minutes before lunch, she had had another insulin injection.

It was clear what a serious impact the diagnosis of diabetes was having on this young child. Diabetes cannot be ignored, no matter how much one tries to set it aside, even for short periods of time. Now that she was home, still weighed down by the pressure she'd been under for so many days, Danai let herself go. I tried to boost her morale and stop her from having destructive thoughts. "Danai," I told her, in a calm, reassuring voice—looking her straight in the eye, "don't ever let anyone in your life make you believe that there is something wrong with you.

Everything happens for a reason," I heard myself telling her.

"And what is the reason for me having diabetes?" she threw out another serious question.

"So that you realize how strong you are!" I said, without stopping to think.

Our discussion ended there. I cannot remember whether I finished lunch or what it tasted like. I don't remember what I did next, or how we left the now awkward and uninviting atmosphere of home and returned to the familiar environment of the hospital. At the hospital, most discussions were about diabetes and ways to cope. We and the staff spoke the same language and did not need to get entangled in superfluous interactions. In the hospital, I did not make unavoidable, automatic comparisons of our life before and after diabetes, although such comparisons followed me everywhere, as soon as I left its grounds. In there, we had never lived a carefree life without diabetes. Diabetes had always been part of our hospital lives, and so I did not have to engage with before and after comparisons.

However, I will never forget that episode on the veranda during lunch. It was a decisive moment for Danai, who accepted my interpretation of current events with a child's wisdom and ability to recognize what was important in life. The thought that the most demanding moments of our lives force us to discover our own powers soothes my soul when I am tested, something that happens often. The answer I gave Danai in response to her big and serious question became the answer to so many of my own "whys."

9. SOMEONE WHO SHOULD NOT BE FORGOTTEN: FIVE-YEAR-OLD IOLI

When one child in a family goes through a difficult time, the parents sometimes pay more attention to that child. This attitude can lead other children in the family to form the false impression that they are not as important to their parents. One of the consequences of such a misinterpretation is that they feel neglected and develop low self-esteem.

Since her birth, Ioli had always been the equal of all other family members. I was careful, especially during this great challenge, to help her feel this even more. Our younger daughter came to the hospital daily after kindergarten and always enjoyed having lunch and spending time with us. At five years old, Ioli also needed to understand what was going on, and why so many things had suddenly changed. She needed to know why her sister was in the hospital, and to accept that children sometimes get sick, needing hospitalization so that doctors can help them. She also needed to feel safe, and to believe that everything would be fine and that soon we would all sleep together under the same roof.

Ioli was very willing to understand and adjusted perfectly to the changes and demands of those days. She adhered to our schedule and accepted my partial absence without objections or complaints. She understood that I needed to spend most nights in the hospital with Danai. Some nights, however, I was able to share with her at home, while her father stayed with Danai. On these occasions, I did something special to reassure her that I was there and had not forgotten her, and that I wanted to take care of her as much as her sister. I filled the tub with water and let her splash and laugh, because this was something that filled her with joy and helped her relax. She too was tired, but, being five years old, was probably not aware of it. A sudden opportunity to splash in the tub and a big hug in the big bed before she fell asleep, were unexpected gifts to Ioli. This was my attempt to make her feel that the world had not turned completely upside down, that part of it had stayed the same. I wanted my younger daughter to believe that she did not have to worry about her sister or anyone else.

Many times, I surprised loli with little gifts to compensate for the upsetting time she was going through. These little gifts were loaded with messages. One day, as she was waiting in the hospital area with her usual exemplary patience, I put a little bracelet around her wrist. She asked why she was receiving so many gifts when it was not her birthday! I let her know that it was my way of showing how much I appreciated her patience and courage, which helped me learn everything I had to know about diabetes. It was important to thank her for helping us face the challenges of that difficult time in our lives, the same challenges that were taking us away from her.

10. WE HAVE TO LEAVE AGAIN

We were approaching the end of Danai's two week stay in the hospital, the short period of time that I initially believed would last an eternity. Naturally, Danai was not the only child needing treatment. During our stay in the hospital we met many children with health problems, some more serious than others. This world, the hospital world, is real in the flesh. It is the other side of the coin we hold in our hands, the coin of life. In all the years before, we had turned a blind eye to this reality. What we experienced before Danai's diagnosis was just one side of the coin. In the hospital world, I met angels: children with chronic diseases who looked directly into my eyes with a zest for life, with eyes that radiated power and an incredible tolerance and bravery, given everything they had to endure. I met children who made me laugh and taught me to show courage, to take strength from their strength.

In a few days, I managed to accomplish what had initially seemed impossible. I was injecting my own child. I learned to estimate the amount of carbohydrates Danai needed to consume, in relation to the amount of insulin she was taking. All of us—Danai, her father, and I— acquired medical knowledge about how the pancreas functions. We knew which changes in that organ caused type one diabetes and how the human body could be affected by various complications. In two weeks, we all (Danai and her parents) became a kind of artificial pancreas, an external intervention regulating the innumerable amazing functions of this wonderful creation of nature. This responsibility filled me not only with awe at the wisdom and perfection with which nature creates and functions, but also with panic and fear at the thought that we could never completely replace the automatic mechanisms nature invented for our survival. I felt that the substitutes we provided (the measuring equipment, syringes, and insulin) were constantly trying to approach the infallibility of the authentic.

Hours before we left the hospital, I experienced something inconceivably human, beneficial, warm, wonderful, and kind. It was given to me completely unexpectedly by a diabetologist, generously and spontaneously, as if from friend to friend. She was one of the doctors who had seen my desperation and fear at first hand during the first minutes and hours after Danai was diagnosed. "Don't worry," she told me, "because of the way you are bringing her up, Danai will make it, she'll be able to leave home and study. She won't have any problems." Her message was that we should not let diabetes dominate our lives or be the center of attention.

She gave me this message just at the moment when I had become convinced that my family's life, and especially Danai's, would always be restricted, with many consequences. I had come to believe that our lives had ended that Monday afternoon at the pediatrician's office, when Danai and I played our final game of hangman, before shouldering the burden of diabetes. I heard the liberating advice of this young doctor, just when I was thinking that it would be almost impossible for us to travel again— and that I would not see Greece for a long time. The doctor's words made me straighten up under the heavy load of the diagnosis.

I knew that, despite having attended intensive hospital classes given by all kinds of specialists over several days, we still had many tasks to accomplish. I knew there was a lot of work ahead of us, less practical than emotional and psychological. The practical side of things doesn't take long to change.

People can adjust to a new reality. However, the way we feel and think require more attention. You have to hammer away at emotional realities in order to progress, evolve, and learn to function in a balanced way. This is especially true when adjusting to staggering events that upset the balance and change the established order of things.

Back then, in the beginning, I did not appreciate that one important step toward achieving psychological balance was to face up to the demands of diabetes and the challenges of our daily routine honestly, genuinely accepting the changes to our familiar way of living. In the swirl of events, I was pushing away the fact that, from that moment onwards, I would have to learn to live in a different way—and most of all that I would have to accept the fact that Danai was diabetic.

When her hospital room was packed up and it was time to leave, I still felt that I did not have the necessary tools to hammer my soul into its new shape. The shock of the diagnosis still affected me. I did not have enough mental power to adjust to it. Accepting my child's condition did not happen automatically. The first days after Danai was diagnosed, I was just surviving. But the young doctor's prediction and advice were valuable tools, encouraging me to think more positively about my child's future. I therefore held them very safe inside me, as a precious treasure. Hours before we left the familiar children's hospital diabetes ward, I held onto this precious gift for the moments ahead when I would need a life jacket to keep from sinking. It became one of the tools that helped me defeat depression.

The fact that I did not immediately accept our new reality was not just because the diagnosis was too harsh, or because events followed one after the other at a crazy pace. Out in the non-diabetic world, I would have to fight with different elements of nature to survive, but right now, my first priority was to monitor the psychological worlds of my children. Focusing on this different and painful reality and struggling to find some balance, I needed much more time. Most of all, I needed isolation. During the first hours and days after we left the hospital, I had neither of those resources.

11. OUR DEPARTURE FROM THE HOSPITAL: THE BIG CHALLENGES BEGIN NOW

We left the hospital, Danai and I, feeling insecure, which made every step feel heavy, as if we were not sure we dared to undertake such a journey. We were leaving the safety of the hospital to face dangers and challenges. What if something happened out there that we couldn't cope with alone? For a moment, it crossed my mind that I would rather stay in the hospital for another couple of months. I was scared of taking on the challenges of diabetes without feeling sure that I was adequately equipped to face them. To expose myself to the non-diabetic world was a dreadful perspective. Outside the hospital, most people had no clue what it meant to live with type one diabetes. I would have to learn to defend and protect myself as well as my children in order to survive.

Danai and I climbed the stairs to our fourth-floor apartment, loaded with all the things we had collected during our two-week hospital stay. Another automatic comparison: two weeks ago, we had left with just one bag—running, panicking, and feeling incredibly upset because the pediatrician had sent us to the hospital as an emergency case and we didn't have the slightest idea what was to follow. Just two weeks later, we walked slowly home, without much energy in reserve. We walked in silence from the car to the building, each of us sunk in her own thoughts, as if trying to postpone the beginning of this new reality—inch by inch and second by second. We walked as if wanting to have the dimensions of space and time on our side, so as not to have to immediately face our new lives, complicated by the demanding responsibilities of diabetes.

That day, returning from the hospital after two weeks, it felt as if we were moving house. Our loot included diabetic equipment—syringes, insulin, spare parts, measuring tapes, books on diabetes—as well as gifts from pharmaceutical companies, teddy bears, clothes, children's books, and visitors' gifts, not to mention the experiences and pictures now imprinted forever in our memories. Of course, we also had the big pink horse, which had lived in Danai's room and would always remind us of the reason for its existence. All of this real and emotional luggage somehow created for me the illusion that we were moving.

Danai and I went into the house where we had lived for years without any idea of what it meant to face the demands of type one diabetes. The sense of the new and unfamiliar made me uncomfortable. In this apartment, which had once been my oasis, and now it no longer felt like home, I felt empty. Now I would have to start all over again, learning to live in this space and getting used to the feeling that it belonged to me. Once again, I had to acclimatize myself to its smells and rooms, until they signaled to me that this was where I could put on my pajamas and rest.

Ioli met us at the door, full of joy that we had finally returned. I understood her reaction—at last, she could have her Mom at home to take care of her and Danai to play with—but I could not share her excitement. It was all I could do to move my body from one point to the next to carry out the day's tasks. I did not want (and was not able) to think very much. Just seconds after we entered the strange, awkward, uninviting space of our home and shut the door behind us, Danai looked at her five-year-old sister and asked, with some frustration, another big question:

"Why should I have diabetes and not her?"

I froze. I felt as if nothing existed but the five-year-old child standing in front of me, on the receiving end of Danai's frustration. Although I was still carrying our luggage from the hospital, I could feel how this comment hurt Ioli, making her feel to blame for everything that had changed in her sister's life. Danai's question snuffed out Ioli's joy at welcoming us home. She turned and looked at me, waiting for an explanation. I had to find a way out of the dead end all three of us were suddenly facing, to intervene and protect this small child from developing negative feelings about herself. Ioli should not feel guilty about the situation Danai was in, as she was not in any way responsible for it.

So, right away, although I did not feel capable of thinking or intervening, I had to act very fast. I said,

"Danai, if someone in a family does not hear well and needs to wear a hearing aid, do you think that everybody else in the family should wear hearing aids too?"

Both children immediately started laughing, forgetting that one was diabetic and the other not. It was a relief to have this issue settled, but later events showed me that this was not the only troublesome thought to sort out for Danai. In the future, diabetes would continue to upset her one way or the other.

We moved on. The next step to take was for all of us to find our places again. We had to start functioning in order to survive. Belongings had to be put away, clothes washed, food cooked, bills paid, and diabetes-related chores and paperwork completed. We also wanted to get back to old habits, like watching TV, playing games, and making phone calls. I had to keep functioning without thinking about how little energy I had for all this, and without letting pain rise to the surface and paralyze me.

Our dinner table was now covered with medical equipment for regulating diabetes. Boxes of syringes, blood sugar measuring tapes, and spare parts—small and bigger boxes—ingredients of a new sort of life. For a few days, I believed this was how we would have to live from now on, and that our table would never be a dinner table again. This idea was upsetting; the thought that we might have to make such a compromise was suffocating.

The advice the thoughtful young doctor had given me just before we left the hospital came to mind: that we should not let diabetes dominate our lives. I was eager to apply this guidance right at the beginning. This precious message gave me a boost to take action faster than I thought I could. I emptied a cupboard filled with maps and travel guides, reference materials for one of our favorite past activities, and filled it with all the diabetes related stuff. Now, at least, the medical supplies would not be constantly on display. We all knew where they were and could find them easily, whenever we needed to.

I felt I had begun to set limits, not only for diabetes but also for myself. We would take care of it without letting it constantly remind us of its existence. We had to teach ourselves (and especially Danai) that life has much more to offer than insulin injections. Putting all of her medical gear into a cupboard and shutting the door lifted a burden from my shoulders. We could use our table for eating and playing board games again, just the way we used to.

In addition to medical equipment, we also had books about treating diabetes. Initially, it upset me to see them lying around the house. Their titles all included the upsetting word, "diabetes," printed in huge, easy-to-read letters. I did not want all of us to be constantly reminded of this condition. I thought of hiding the books so that no one would look at them, not just my family, but also visitors. Then I stopped and reconsidered. Was it right to indulge this sort of self-delusion? What sort of message would it send to the children—especially Danai—if I hid the books away? Was diabetes a condition to be afraid or ashamed of? Should she learn to deny its permanency? Stopping to think made me realize that my initial reaction had been simply to escape. I wanted to deny the reality of diabetes and its permanent character in our lives. I did not want to believe that my daughter was really affected; subconsciously, I thought that, by hiding books meant to teach us about the peculiarities of diabetes, I would be able to stop thinking about it.

A very quick self-analysis showed me that I was trying to create an illusion, despite understanding that illusions are merely fake sensations. The truth may be unbearable, but it has an authenticity and nobleness that illusions lack. They are second-class sensations, a cheap substitute for the truth—fragile, and ready to betray you at any moment. On the other hand, if you open your arms to the truth, sooner or later it will compensate you. The truth empowers you and equips you to face challenges. Something like that happened when I decided not to hide the diabetes books. I felt I was becoming stronger, as I squeezed them between children's books about different kinds of horses, a history of the Olympic Games, animal babies, and a thousand dolls and their stories. I stood in front of the bookshelves and looked at our collection of books. Yes, that was where the books on diabetes belonged. Denying them would be like denying the existence of my child, who was now diabetic. Nothing hurt as much as that last thought.

Not even the knowledge that Danai now had diabetes.

12. DANAI FACES NEW CHALLENGES

The fact that I kept the diabetes books in public view did not, of course, mean the end of our tribulations. Home from the hospital, Danai now faced a paradox: she had to continue being a child, while at the same time, she was robbed of her childhood. She found herself caught between two worlds: the old familiar, carefree, happy, hilarious, and absolutely childlike world and the new, cruel, austere, painful, and demanding world of diabetes. She was forced to mix old and new realities and to accept her new identity for the sake of survival.

In just two weeks, inconceivably fast, this eight-year-old girl was expected to integrate a new world into the already existing one. Danai, her clothes still smelling of the hospital and her ears full of the voices of doctors telling her how much insulin to inject and food to consume, found herself home and faced with a huge task: to stab her fingers many times a day to measure the levels of sugar in her blood and estimate the quantity of carbohydrates she needed to eat. She also had to accept that she could eat only at specific times, regardless of how hungry she felt. In addition, she had to tolerate many injections of insulin, all through the day and night and carefully observe her body's messages, interpret them in the right way, and act accordingly. As an eight-year-old child, Danai had to be able to detect the symptoms of hypoglycemia and respond fast, in order to avoid a dangerous and unpleasant situation. She also had to go on living—getting ready for school, meeting her friends, watching TV, playing with her sister, going to the movies, and taking part in family excursions.

From now on, Danai would have to navigate through life with a new map. When we came home from the hospital, this huge life change made me realize what it would mean for her to carry such a heavy load on her shoulders. In her familiar environment, Danai's attitude towards diabetes changed considerably. The need to adjust so suddenly to the new situation was beyond her capacity. At home she behaved very differently than she had in the hospital. She stopped trying to control her feelings. Although we never discussed it, I believe that she too found it impossible to be home without making comparisons, if only unconsciously. I cannot otherwise explain her succession of reactions and her unwillingness to cooperate when it came to diabetes.

In the hospital, nothing much happens other than doctors examining you and nurses giving you injections. You expect injections in the hospital, but not in your own home. At home, there is no medical staff coming in and out of your room to examine you, no machines making noises all night long, no children crying, and no one stabbing your fingers to measure your blood sugar levels. At home, you eat and sleep as much as you want, without anyone waking you up to measure your sugar levels in your blood or ordering you to drink juice in the middle of the night. At home, you invite friends over, jump rope, and run and laugh. You don't have to sit on the sidelines because you feel weak and shivery and can't see well enough to participate.

Once, at a meeting with other diabetic families and doctors, specialists told us the estimated number of injections that a diabetic child has to put up within a year. The number was so shocking that I made the deliberate decision not to store it in my memory. I was experiencing the adventure of diabetes first hand; I had a vague notion of how many needles would stab my child's body every year but did not want to form a precise picture of the situation with the help of mathematical calculations. These unavoidable thousands of injections are preceded by even more thousands of unavoidable blood sugar measurements. The fingers are used for that purpose, suffering multiple needle invasions.

Injections became part of Danai's life suddenly, at a moment of crisis, just as diabetes had. While in the hospital she'd been willing from the start to inject the insulin herself, at home she abandoned this cooperative attitude. As a result, the issue of injections (with all it entailed) was becoming more and more complicated and difficult to handle. Danai's body and soul intensely objected to injections, an attitude that lasted for more than four years. During that whole time, she not only refused to inject the insulin herself, she also lived in agony. She often panicked at the sight of the syringe, while many pierced her body daily. Often, she categorically refused to acknowledge that the injections were even necessary, regardless of who was trying to inject her.

Thousands of needles stabbed into Danai's hips and thighs during this four-year period. Although they were really tiny, they still were an artificial body penetrating a human one. The marks the needles made were visible as well as tangible. Her skin was bruised and often hard; this made Danai detest the mandatory piercing even more. Each time, we had to search for a spot that would work for the next injection. The bruises and changes to her body did not give us many options. The pain caused by insulin spreading under her skin was also a factor, perhaps causing more discomfort than the needles did.

I interpret this behavior as the result of the child being back in her safe home, where most things were allowed. At home, she felt comfortable and free to express herself without worrying about the impression she made on others. Perhaps in the hospital the presence of so many strangers forced her to suppress her true feelings and made her follow orders without any objections. I did not want to put Danai under pressure by asking her to explain her different reactions at home and in the hospital. I chose to keep my observations and interpretations of her behavior to myself.

As a type one diabetic, unless you use an insulin pump, you have to inject insulin wherever you are: at home, in the car, at the airport, in fields or zoos, at parties, on boats, in offices, factories and forests, at school and kindergarten, in restaurants and in taxis, on beaches and at taverns, in airplanes, and even on hot air balloons. Insulin injections are not a matter of choice, they are mandatory: a matter of life and death. As time passed, I began to get over my own psychological pain whenever Danai injected insulin, especially when she refused and had to be persuaded to do it. My maternal instincts made me realize that I had to be her prop, the one who made her feel strong. For this reason, I moved towards the opposite pole, focusing on helping her get through the whole injection process faster and with as little pain as possible.

As time passed, in order to be able to deal with the demands of diabetes, I learned not to concentrate so much on feelings, either my own or Danai's, but to approach the whole process with a somewhat professional attitude, like a nurse. I learned to distance myself. I could not afford to let daily friction or mental pain wear me down. I had to create conditions that would give me enough energy to meet the demands, not only of Danai's diabetes, but also of the rest of my daily routine.

I invented a number of different ways to convince Danai to have her insulin injection. I sometimes took a syringe and stuck it into my own thigh to prove that injections weren't painful if done at the right speed. I explained that the needle was tiny and nothing to be afraid of. I also encouraged her not to focus on the actual injection every time, on the needle penetrating her body and the possibility of feeling pain, but to think instead about her favorite beach in Greece, or about the pink paws of her tomcat, or the nice time we were going to have on our next planned escape. Our brains, I told her, can only process one piece of information at a time; if she occupied her mind with a positive thought at the moment of injection, she would not feel pain, or at least not to the extent she expected to. Danai, depending on her mood, could not always follow this piece of advice, but whenever she did, she was rewarded with a less traumatic ritual.

Meanwhile, we frequently had to deal with criticism from others, who complained that we were parenting Danai in the wrong way. Every two or three months, we went back to the hospital for a routine checkup with the diabetologist responsible for Danai, and every time he asked whether she had started to inject herself. When we said that she hadn't, he asked Danai's age, which he already knew, implying that she was old enough to do it. He treated this issue as one of the most important problems he had to solve. We also met mothers of other diabetic children, who enjoyed comparing their cases to ours. These mothers always mentioned their own children's exemplary behavior in injecting insulin from a very early age, implying that we did not understand how to care for or deal with our child.

In my life, I have learned to appreciate the diversity of human nature and I have always encouraged my children to just be themselves. Moreover, I try at every available opportunity to teach my daughters the importance of learning to trust their own instincts. Deciding whether or not to inject insulin gave Danai a chance to practice this approach and cultivate this valuable tool. The right time for her to start injecting insulin was when she felt it was the right time.

Amidst all these turbulent events and the feelings they aroused, it would be wrong to ignore the effect diabetes had on loli. Our five-year-old also experienced the tension and drama of Danai's daily insulin injections, as well as the other stresses of life with type one diabetes. She absorbed Danai's reactions and ours so intensely that she even offered to give the insulin injection to Danai herself, perhaps hoping to resolve the issue fast. Such moments were a good opportunity to remind loli that the treatment of diabetes was not her responsibility, just as she was not responsible for Danai's feelings.

Danai's attitude toward injecting insulin changed during a quarrel with me. I pointed out that one way to become more independent was to be brave enough to manage her own injections. It was the right moment, a moment of liberation, not only for Danai but also for me. This change was a welcome step towards more freedom of movement and independence for her. It was a step towards more freedom of movement and independence for me as well.

13. GOING BACK TO SCHOOL AND FACING NEW CHALLENGES, FEARS, AND MISTAKES

Another burden, which added to the turmoil we experienced daily after leaving the hospital, was Danai's return to school. Before she was diagnosed with diabetes, our main challenge of the morning was to get her out of bed on time, and to make sure she was dressed and finished with breakfast before it was time to walk up the hill to school. After the hospital, Danai's morning insulin injection became a stressful new part of this ritual, needing to be overcome in a creative and resourceful manner. All of us faced an unprecedented challenge. Diabetes had the power of a tornado pulling us away—we had to find something to hold on to tightly, so as not to be sucked into the whirlwind.

This new situation and sequence of events took a toll on our daily routine. None of the three of us, neither Danai nor her parents, were initially able to manage this challenge with poise. The very first mornings home from the hospital were critically important and we needed to face them calmly, something we did not always succeed in doing. Everything had to happen fast, as school wouldn't wait and time never stops. Classes begin with or without you. After the hospital, it wasn't enough to shout, as we used to: "Get dressed quickly! Drink your milk, we have to go!" Now we had to convince an eight-year-old child to allow us to stab her body with a needle before she had even opened her eyes. A child who reacted, resisted, protested, and certainly detested what she was forced to tolerate, day in and day out.

Every day, early in the morning, every movement had to be strictly coordinated so that Danai would not be late for school. The pressure on all three of us—not only time pressure but also psychological pressure— made us relate badly to each other. It was essential for us to show empathy and express care, introducing humor even into such demanding circumstances; this accelerated the whole process and made it less painful for Danai. However, the emotional charge and time pressure made it hard to remember that threats and tension had no place in a child's room. Pressure made it difficult to remember how unproductive it was to panic exactly at the moment when Danai needed reassurance and special care. When we did manage to adopt a strategy that reinforced the efforts Danai was making to cope with the horrific demands of diabetes—and whenever we praised her for being so brave—the ordeal of the morning insulin injection was completed faster.

During this ordeal, our way of life was changing and not for the better. Our fears and the struggle to accept reality, the control we exercised over our resourceful child, and the exhaustion and sleeping disorders caused by frequent nighttime blood measurements led us into a psychological dead end comprised of mental pain, helplessness, sorrow, and desperation. The permanence of the new reality, as well as the extent of its demands, tested everyone in the family, and most of all, of course, Danai. Whether we liked it or not, we had to face it with discipline and meet its demands promptly, with no deviations. The Spartan discipline imposed by diabetes exercised enormous pressure on us. Our decreasing freedom of movement made me feel that our living space was getting smaller—shrinking like a piece of cloth after washing, and preventing me from being the person I wanted to be.

The new living conditions pushed us to our limits on a daily basis. We disagreed with one another and blamed each other for our mistakes. Each one of us knew the best way to make injections less upsetting; each one of us knew the best way to regulate diabetes, and of course our shared secret was that none of us wanted to live with it.

After experimenting with different ways of dealing with injections, we concluded that I should take over the morning sessions. As the needle entered Danai's body, I would distract her with interesting discussions, talking about topics that had nothing to do with diabetes. The sooner this ritual was over, the less painful it would be. Over time, our tensions, fears, and panic reactions significantly lessened but did not vanish. More experience made us realize that it was even better to give the morning injection while Danai was still asleep. Ioli was of course a permanent observer and part of the whole situation.

As soon as we had accomplished the first part of our morning preparations for school, the second part was waiting. Like every other stage, it had to be executed with absolute precision. Every morning, Danai had to have in her school bag a snack box containing the exact amount of carbohydrates she needed to consume at school at a specific time, corresponding to the amount of insulin we'd injected her with before she left home. Before Danai left home to go anywhere, we had to make sure that she carried with her everything she needed to survive diabetes. The first few times I made her snack, I had to tell myself that I was not allowed to cry—at least not with visible tears. I let my inner self cry as much as it wanted to, since no one could see invisible tears. I did not want the children to know how much the new turn of events was hurting me.

Before Danai was diagnosed with diabetes, she walked with her friends up the hill to school every morning, with her school bag on her back. We can all imagine such moments, when children share news of the previous day and talk with friends about ordinary school fears and joys before the start of class. Such moments were erased from Danai's daily routine. She stopped meeting her friends around the corner and sharing their first encounters of the day. After her diagnosis, she stopped walking up the hill. The fear that this physical activity could cause her to become hypoglycemic forced us to drive her to school every morning.

Every day, we left Danai in the schoolyard with her unpredictable diabetes, not knowing how her body would react to the insulin she had received, or to physical activity, stress, or the carbohydrates she would consume later. Every morning, we left Danai alone with her diabetes, knowing that it would force her body to function according to its rules, and that she would have to religiously observe its reactions and demands.

As soon as Danai was no longer under our supervision, she was exposed to greater risks. Every morning, when we left her at school, we felt insecure, worrying that she might not be able to cope with the demands of school life, or that she might not measure her blood sugar levels on time, or have enough food to meet her physical needs. Her classmates knew to keep an eye on her reactions. The girlfriends she spent her breaks with had candy in their bags and knew they had to run and get help if they had any suspicion that Danai's behavior had changed. Danai was the only child in her class who was allowed to eat at any time, wherever she was, even during class. When other children brought sweets to school for their birthdays, only Danai was left out. When her teacher bought ice cream for the class, she had to go without—not because it was sweet (an obsolete rule for diabetics), but because (like most treats) it was offered outside her strict eating timetable. Moreover, she was the only child who needed to measure her blood sugar and rest when suffering from hypoglycemia, or to inject insulin during school excursions.

While Danai was at school, we carefully planned the rest of the day. Lunch had to be cooked and ready to be served the moment she came home at lunchtime.

This was so tightly scheduled that, when we picked her up at school in the car, we had to follow the same route home each time, without even the option of stopping off somewhere else for a few minutes. We had to minimize the possibility of Danai getting hypoglycemic and be ready to treat her for a possible hypoglycemic episode at lunchtime. When classes ended, she was immediately spirited home, discreetly but very quickly. She could never go home with her friends the way she used to, carefree and relaxed. She missed all of their chats about what had happened at school and who was visiting whom. She could not unwind and converse with other kids, while walking down the hill at the end of the day.

On the Friday of Danai's first week back at school, it was time for her swimming class, just as it had been on that critical Friday when her teacher noticed her getting tired suspiciously fast. The day he had told Danai to ask her parents to take her to the doctor had been just three weeks earlier; psychological time ticks differently. For eight-year-old Danai, that swimming class had become the cause of her diabetes diagnosis. She believed that, if her teacher had not sent her to the doctor, the following three weeks of trauma would never have happened.

That first Friday back was completely different from the time before. She would be swimming after receiving a lower than usual dose of insulin, escorted by her father, who would monitor her measurements, and make sure she had the right amount of juice or carbohydrates to avoid becoming hypoglycemic while swimming. Danai was the only child in her class for whom low blood sugar levels meant that she had to get out of the water to manage her needs, even if that completely interrupted her swimming. At the same time, she would watch her friends splashing in the water, feeling carefree and safe, with no idea what it was like to live with diabetes.

Danai entered the swimming pool that day afraid that she would not be able to do it, and that she might feel the same exhaustion she had experienced the day her teacher had made her get out of the water. She stepped into the pool afraid that she might drown. That first swimming class was a day of fear for her. She had recently learned what it feels like when your own body betrays you, when there is no energy left to keep you going. She had not forgotten how her weakness had scared her when she was swimming in deep water. In this way, Danai's favorite activity had become a life-threatening and dangerous situation, completely unappealing to her. For a long period of time after her diagnosis, she refused to go swimming with us. It took a lot of work for her to stop thinking of swimming as a life-threatening situation, or associating it with diabetes and its symptoms. She had to practice having new experiences in water, time after time, in order to feel secure and to stop being afraid that she would drown. Eventually, she became a confident swimmer again and her traumatic memories began to fade away. The support she received from my husband and me gave her the chance to erase unpleasant memories and replace them with new, more pleasant and positive experiences. Her courage was rewarded with moments of joy and action, almost like old times.

During mandatory school track and field activities, Danai could not be unaccompanied during the first weeks after her diagnosis. I spent hours on the sports field worrying about whether she would be able to run without causing her blood sugar levels to drop dangerously. Although she was given less insulin and consumed additional carbohydrates before each physical activity, we could never be sure that these extra precautions would be effective. Multiple factors influence the concentration of sugar in the blood, making it impossible to achieve desirable blood sugar levels at every moment of the day and night.

Life's demands, such as school performances or sports competitions, can impact the course of diabetes. This situation made me feel as if the condition could easily slip from our control, as a fish slips through the fisherman's fingers. Although my presence at the sports field was necessary in the beginning of our symbiosis with type one diabetes, our relationship depended on my monitoring her in a discreet way. I hit upon a method that involved using cell phones to remind Danai from a distance what she needed to do to avoid hypoglycemia. We thus achieved an effective way of cooperating that didn't trigger comments or awkward feelings.

It was fundamental for Danai to realize that, setting aside her additional responsibilities as a diabetic, she was still able to take part in school activities. I remember her on that sunny day not being any different from the other children. I remember the positive contribution she made to her team, with her talent for movement and coordination. She was integrated into the group, not marginalized or stigmatized. Such moments offered important reasons to feel happy, then and in the future. On that particular sunny day of school track and field activities, our whole family received a hopeful message: diabetes, provided that you take good care of it, does not present an obstacle to new experiences or obstruct a person's zeal for action and creativity. Danai's ability to adapt to her new life—her willingness to be part of it—was more important than the risk of becoming hypoglycemic.

School life carried on, but not in the usual way. Each new day that we survived the machinations of diabetes felt like a day when we accomplished something special. Before we left the hospital, all of the staff at Danai's school had been told about the new turn our life had taken. Up to then, none of the teachers had ever received any information on how to deal with the emergencies a diabetic child could face. The school director told us that a diabetic child had attended the school once before, but the staff had not learned about the demands of diabetes and would not have known how to react in an emergency.

When a hospital counselor offered to brief the teachers at Danai′s school, and particularly Danai′s teacher, the offer was rejected without a convincing explanation. No one at school thought it was important to invest time—either to learn what diabetes type one could mean, or how to respond in an emergency. At this point, it is worth mentioning that the school is within walking distance of the hospital, so no one ever had to drive there through heavy traffic wasting time or losing his or her temper, as is usually the case in big cities. It is also worth mentioning that the hospital counselor told school staff that the information session would last for just one hour and be free of charge. Despite these ideal learning conditions, every teacher and the school administrator rejected the hospital's offer flat out, showing complete indifference to the prospect of learning some basic information about diabetes. This negative attitude made my husband and me feel even more insecure when Danai was away from home.

The person who spent the most hours with Danai on a daily basis was her teacher. It was highly probable that she would eventually face an emergency, without being able to respond appropriately. The scale of indifference that her teacher demonstrated (despite being mainly responsible for Danai's safety) confirmed my impression that she was unsuitable for this job. The consequences of this attitude did not take long to manifest. One morning, just a few days after Danai's return to school, my phone rang while I was in the supermarket. After my daughter's diagnosis, I overcame my dislike of phones and always carried one with me, its battery always charged. I knew exactly which trouser pocket it was in, so that I never had to waste valuable time looking for it before answering a call that could be related to Danai's needs.

That day, one child was at school and the other at kindergarten. When I answered the call, the shrill voice of this amazing pedagogue shook me to the core. Danai was having some sort of crisis! Something was wrong with her heart and I had to get to school fast, she told me. I dropped my basket of shopping and started running through the aisles, past the cash tills, and outside, reaching the car in a flash. I got to Danai's school as fast as I could, driving through town at high speed. If the police had chosen that moment to ask me to stop, they would have seen me parking half on the pavement outside the school gate, and running like a fugitive through the glass door towards my daughter's class.

When I arrived, I found Danai standing out in the schoolyard with her body shaking, having difficulties breathing. I could not figure out what was going on— whether she was shaking because her teacher had let her stay out in the cold without her jacket, or whether she was afraid for her life. This amazing pedagogue announced to me that Danai had felt unwell during a test, and so she had sent her to an empty room next door, where she would not "disturb the other children." Even worse, Danai's teacher had forced her to eat without asking her to measure her blood sugar levels first.

I had warned this cold-blooded woman, while Danai was still in the hospital, that no one should pity her when she came back to school. I remember emphasizing that she did not have to show any pity to my child, knowing her abrupt and inappropriate behavior towards children. I wanted to protect Danai from becoming embroiled in various traumatic scenarios. I had not thought it would be necessary to explain to this teacher the importance of paying attention to Danai's condition to avert emergencies, or to make sure that she was never left alone in an empty room, especially when she wasn't feeling well. I could not have believed how indifferent this teacher would prove to be, just a few days later, when faced with Danai's special needs. Her mismanagement of this emergency made the eight-year-old's condition deteriorate so quickly that she panicked. I drove her very quickly to the hospital, still in a state of panic, while all the time trying to reassure her that everything would be fine and her life was not in danger.

I parked right outside the hospital door (illegally) to find medical help as fast as possible. By this time, Danai was telling me that she could not feel her legs or walk. I carried her into the hospital shouting that I had an emergency: this child needed a diabetologist immediately! Help came fast. The doctor who examined her concluded that Danai could not have become hypoglycemic at school, judging from her blood sugar values at the hospital. Her symptoms must have been caused by something else and should never have been treated without measuring the level of sugar in Danai's blood, a fast and easy process.

Her teacher's reaction had been completely wrong and dangerous. After the doctors stabilized my daughter's condition, we went home and analyzed the situation to figure out what had caused the problem. Danai had been taking a test when she felt her heart beating quickly. Not being able yet to correctly interpret psychosomatic symptoms, she had jumped to the conclusion that there was something wrong with her heart. Anxiety exacerbated the problem and her physical reactions made her panic. She was caught in a vicious circle that sent her back to the hospital.

During her early encounters with diabetes, Danai shouldered the huge responsibility of having to learn to observe her own physical reactions with great precision, while at the same time evaluating and correctly interpreting the messages her organism was sending her. The young and inexperienced child was not always able to do this. Many times, hypoglycemia symptoms made her panic, feel very afraid, and exaggerate the perilousness of her situation. She remembered having a cardiogram at the pediatrician's office and perhaps that was one of the reasons why she associated her symptoms with heart problems. I had to reassure her repeatedly that the rapid beating of her heart did not mean there was anything wrong with it, as her recent cardiogram had proved. I suggested visiting the pediatrician again to convince her that her symptoms had been caused by hypoglycemia and nothing else. She refused. Visits to doctors had to be kept to an absolute minimum. After many discussions about the condition of her heart, Danai preferred to trust my reassurances, rather than face another doctor or medical examination.

Shaking, another symptom of hypoglycemia, made it harder for her to adjust to her new condition. It terrified and unsettled her, making her constantly worry about her own life, and doubt whether she could manage to survive away from home. Days after Danai's diagnosis, the simple act of going to the playground, a natural ingredient of life before diabetes, transformed into a repulsive activity. It was interpreted by her as a threat that could cause hypoglycemia. Even if we got there, she refused to run between the swings and the seesaw, or from the seesaw to the jungle gym. Eventually, she stopped engaging in active play altogether.

Because Danai had experienced repeated episodes of hypoglycemia after physical activity, it was sometimes impossible to motivate or persuade her to leave the house. We often cancelled plans to go out when Danai chose the safety of the couch at home instead of an opportunity to live like a child or have an adventure. I saw her becoming insecure and knew that she believed she couldn't manage physical activities without her blood sugar dropping to dangerous levels. I assumed that she was remembering what had happened the last time she dared to behave like an ordinary child. I saw fear in her eyes at the thought of going through that experience again.

Danai's negative attitude toward life lifted one day, when I took advantage of a moment when my own hands were shaking because I had forgotten to eat. When I showed her the impact my own diet had on me, I noticed her feeling of satisfaction at not being the only person in the world with shaking hands. I could tell that she was beginning to realize that her own symptoms were not alien, and that even her

Mom's hands could tremble, from a kind of hypoglycemic reaction.

Despite multiple reassurances that the symptoms were caused by low levels of sugar in her blood, Danai's negative state of mind did not improve overnight. It took a long time and many discussions, undertaken with compassion, patience, and some humor, for her to find the courage to make her own observations and start to believe that her life was not under threat. With time, her panic attacks, fears, and worries about having a heart condition became less frequent, until they finally disappeared. Responding to her emotional needs and giving her time to learn to interpret her body's messages in the right way, while sharing her pain and a sense of togetherness, provided a form of therapy that got Danai off the couch.

14. THE RETURN TO FAMILIAR, PLEASANT ACTIVITIES

After the adventure of Danai's diagnosis, it was important for the children to return to familiar, pleasant activities of the past. They needed to go back to their extracurricular activities: dance class on Mondays and horseback riding on Fridays. Danai attended dance class three days after leaving the hospital. At her dance school, parents could either choose to wait in the reception area while their children were in class, or take advantage of the free time to go to the supermarket, jog, or do anything they wanted in the short interval available to them. Danai started dancing when she was four years old, four years before being diagnosed with diabetes type one. All through those years, that hour of dance tuition for Danai and Ioli had provided a small oasis for my body and mind. It was time I spent relaxing, reading, drinking tea, or listening to the stories of the other parents (mainly mothers) who shared the room with me.

The day Danai returned to dance class was our first day out of the house after coming home from the hospital. When I entered that familiar space filled with pleasant memories, the comparisons began to torture me once more. On our last visit, we hadn't had the slightest idea what would happen just a few days later. Danai was not diabetic then, or at least we did not know that she was. She did not measure her blood sugar or need insulin injections—and all this was only three weeks earlier! Although the furnishings of the reception area had not changed, I felt (as in so many other familiar places) that everything was different. It did not help that the big plants and bamboo chairs, the bench with tea cups, the black and white pictures of dancers hanging on the walls, the old piano, carpets, changing rooms, and smells remained exactly the same as they'd been for the past four years. Everything seemed very different and almost confusing, because my whole world was turned upside down. In the dance school during class, before Danai was diagnosed with diabetes, I used to feel wonderful; now I felt devastated and empty. Deep inside, I wished I could keep forever what my children and I had shared in the room before the diagnosis of diabetes; the fact that I could not was shattering.

Danai changed into her dance outfit and went to class. So did Ioli. Some of the parents who had dropped off their children were already leaving. The voices, the black and pink outfits, the heads of children bouncing as they rushed to get ready and make it to class on time, all this movement and sound gradually faded out of the corridor until the place where I was standing turned much quieter. I could only hear from a distance, through closed doors, the voices of teachers and the music the children were dancing to. Suddenly, a thought crossed my mind that made me freeze: what if Danai became hypoglycemic?

I trembled at the thought that something could go wrong and prevent her from participating in class. I was not fanatical about her dancing, but I did not want her to feel inhibited or start thinking that she could not continue her favorite activities because of diabetes. I had to stay put. I was there for her if she needed me. Minutes later, the director of the school came out of her office.

"I need to talk to you," I told her.

"I know," she replied.

I had known her for years and we had a good formal relationship. I wanted to talk to her about the peculiar situation we had suddenly found ourselves in as a family. I wanted to make sure that Danai's dance teacher knew to look out for the signs of hypoglycemia. The dance school director already knew about the diagnosis because a friend of Danai's had talked to their teacher, who in turn had talked to the director.

She suggested that we have a private conversation in her office. Our issue was serious and very personal and I did not want spectators, so I welcomed her offer. Sobbing, I described the events of the past two weeks. My automatic reaction of making comparisons returned to torture me. A few days ago, everything had been carefree. My daughter had been able to dance without either of us worrying about her stamina. The director tried to encourage me by saying that everything would turn out well, and I shouldn't worry. Danai's teacher had already been told and would respond right away if she needed to. The director went to look for tissues to dry my tears. My reserves were exhausted.

While I was narrating our adventure, waves of negative emotion came to the surface again, uninvited, hitting me with their familiar, ruthless force. I remember feeling unbearably sad, as if my body were bent under pain. I also felt disadvantaged. My child's condition was not transient. I could not bear the thought that Danai would have to live such a difficult life. I felt that I had lost a battle—a mother's fight to preserve the physical integrity of her children. Any amount of compassion was welcome and helpful.

I heard the director telling me that she was there to support us and would be happy to do so. She helped me by patting me on the shoulder, spending time listening, and sympathizing with my pain. We needed all kinds of help and I did not reject any offers. One hour passed as if it had been a minute. Through the director's office door, I started to hear the voices of children coming out of dance classes into the changing rooms and getting ready to go home.

Dance teachers came into the office one after another. One of them, an American, joined our discussion when she heard me say that I could not stand the thought that Danai had inherited diabetes through me, because my father was diabetic. This American dancer rushed to tell me that her sister, who was a pediatrician, had diagnosed diabetes type one in her own son without being able to trace any other diabetics in her family for many generations. Her nephew could not have inherited diabetes from anyone in his family.

This information dried some of my tears. The rest I did myself. I appreciated the contact with those two women. I will never forget that moment—how relieved I felt to be able to share my pain, knowing that someone empathic and caring was there for me. The moment did not last long, but it worked like a balm on my tormented psyche. Unfortunately, although our discussion was therapeutic and the women's compassion and encouragement made my load lighter, I still had to leave all this and face cruel reality once more. Every minute after that dance class was critical. We had to rush home. No deviations were allowed. There wasn't enough time even to stop briefly at the bakery. Our new, fixed routine had to be followed religiously. I had to make sure we got home on time for dinner and the next dose of insulin and blood sugar measurement.

Since that Monday dance class under the shadow of diabetes, there have been days that have not been easy for Danai. The way she felt physically as well as emotionally fluctuated more than before, impacting her daily schedule to a considerable degree. However, it was very important for her to continue to take part in activities she enjoyed, including dancing. We unfailingly followed the doctor's advice: the gift I had received before we left the hospital. We refused to let diabetes dominate our lives or radically change them.

The next challenge was a favorite activity for many girls: horseback riding. No amount of difficulty or special needs could come between Danai and her passion for horses. So, as soon as we had a chance after leaving the hospital, we drove out to the stables to give the children a chance to do something they loved, and to forget (at least for a while) the hardships of the recent past. It was a difficult contrast: that summer, just days before the pediatrician had sent us to the diabetes ward of the children's hospital, Danai and Ioli had participated in a course on caring for horses. Together with other children, they had cleaned stables and shoveled hay, working from nine in the morning until six in the afternoon, with very few short breaks. Every morning, I had taken the children to the stables with their lunch boxes, and every late afternoon, I had picked them up. I remember finding Danai dirty but cheerful, at peace with the world, and absolutely satisfied at having had so many hours to be close to and care for the animals she adored.

Now, one diagnosis later, she was under the influence of injected insulin and every movement she made had to be monitored. She restricted herself to taking riding lessons; we had to see how her body would react. To stay longer at the stables or do anything other than ride was risky now and could cause her to become hypoglycemic. Either my husband or I had to be present at all times, counting the minutes she was physically active and hoping that the extra carbohydrates she had consumed before the activity, as a precaution, would be enough to sustain her and help her escape complications. The comparison between the past and the present rose to the surface again, as painful as always.

How would I feel if I had to have bodyguards constantly beside me, constantly reminding me to prick my fingers and measure my blood sugar levels? That thought alone was troubling. How must an eight-year-old child feel, when so many things had changed so suddenly since her last visit to the stables? Our omnipresence, like a huge mobile alarm clock, did nothing to boost her morale. However, it was the best compromise we could all make to accommodate the demands of diabetes and horseback riding.

Danai's teacher was clearly bewildered. What was all this about? Why did we constantly supervise our daughter—timing her, and insisting that she eat? Why did we restrict her movement, and what were we all so worried about? Welcome to the world of diabetes, of insulin injections, blood sugar measurements, and hypoglycemia. I can sympathize with the reaction of outsiders. Life with diabetes is a very peculiar and complicated affair. Unless you cross the threshold yourself, you will never really feel its magnitude or understand its dynamics.

Back then, we were beginners. The steps we took in our new life with diabetes were small and very careful. In time, we learned to adjust the needs of this condition to the needs of horseback riding in a more efficient way. Less insulin and more carbohydrates helped to reduce the risk of hypoglycemia. We did not always manage to balance the needs of Danai's body with the demands of her life, but at least we were never defeated by the frustrations of diabetes. The experience we acquired, day by day, gave us confidence and the knowledge that, as long as we remembered to bring all of the diabetic equipment, we could plan more outings and have experiences that would make diabetes and its demands a secondary issue.

In time, we grew more and more distant from the diabetologists of the hospital who were often unavailable when we needed them the most, and called to get their advice. Experience and common sense enabled us to solve problems faster and more efficiently. Dealing successfully with various demands and conditions diabetes imposed on us, boosted our confidence and showed us that we could become more independent.

Gradually, we integrated the peculiarities of diabetes into our lives and, with appropriate planning, began to go on smaller and larger expeditions. More and more often, we set out on new adventures and enjoyed the fun of travelling, always taking with us syringes, insulin in a special cool pack, measuring equipment and replacement needles, food, juice, and candy, a lot of courage and strength, and the awareness that we did not want to live a shrunken life.

One of the bigger challenges we overcame was risking a trip to Greece for Christmas, only four months after Danai's admission to the hospital. It was our first Christmas with diabetes, and we took the risk partly to prove to ourselves that its demands wouldn't drag us down. Danai's doctors encouraged us to follow through with our plans, and reassured us that we would be able to solve any major problems that arose with the help of Greek specialists. Before we left, I did some research and found out whom I could turn to in Athens if we faced a particularly difficult situation.

When we arrived at the airport, I felt the way I always did in familiar places. Still plagued with automatic comparisons, I felt that nothing was the same, even though everything still looked the same. Despite the courage we had demonstrated in travelling so far from home, I agonized over whether we would be able to manage Danai's diabetes, given the schedule of our flight to Athens. One way to make it work was to bring with us not just emergency provisions but also a meal that she could eat at the right time for her scheduled dose of insulin.

Another thing that worried me was the hand luggage restrictions. I thought that we might face special problems, as we were carrying all kinds of items for the care of diabetes. I did not know how the airport personnel would react to the contents of our bags. The little card that I first saw in the office of Mrs. In-a-Hurry, which had made me panic and shudder with its alarming message, "diabetic in need of help," was now in Danai's pouch as a valuable document, to prove that we had a reason for carrying everything we had. Naturally, Danai was planning to show it to the person in charge of luggage.

Surprise number one: the person in charge did not ask to see any documents. He just inquired discreetly which one of us was diabetic; we told him in the same discreet way. Surprise number two: none of the luggage handlers carried out a thorough examination of their contents. Nobody wanted to see more than they had to. They did not want to see the insulin and they did not ask questions or expect answers. They let us right through, as if there were no standard safety regulations on the liquids allowed in airplanes. They did not even search the special bag we used to carry insulin.

This experience gave us wings. If this was how airport staff, who otherwise checked handbags very thoroughly for liquids, treated a diabetic child, then I could only conclude that millions of diabetics had passed through this checkpoint. I felt joy and relief, not only because our courage had been rewarded, but also because I suddenly felt we were not alone in the world of diabetes. Who could say how many other people in that one airport were travelling with insulin? Who could say how many of the people around us belonged to our world? Our first trip with diabetes was less complicated than I had expected. The fear that overcame me a few hours after Danai's diagnosis—that we would not be able to travel anymore and that I would not see Greece for many years—began fading away at that moment. Because we dared to try a major trip, putting our new situation to the test, we gained the confidence to embark on more adventures. Ice skating in Athens, here we come!

And we did come. It was a period when ice skating was becoming very popular in Athens around Christmastime. Many Greeks were putting on skates and attempting to stand and slide on the ice for the first time. We found a beautiful spot at the Port of Faliro to try out this sport. If you have never tried ice skating, you might think it was an easy, relaxing activity, and that you just have to stand and let the icy surface move you along. However, balancing on smooth ice with blades under your feet is exhausting; it makes you sweat even at low temperatures.

At the Port of Faliro, we had to let Danai feel the joy of movement; we could hear Christmas music over megaphones, mingled with the voices of excited people enjoying a new and festive activity. The atmosphere was fantastic. Happy faces, movement, lights, and laughter were all around us, set against the tranquility of the sea and a collection of private yachts that reminded us of summer vacations, a welcome contrast. Everyone around us seemed to be enjoying the experience without having to worry about every move they made. However, my husband and I were on the alert. On the one hand, we wanted Danai to forget her worries in this festive atmosphere, but on the other hand, we ourselves could not forget them for a minute. We were constantly calculating, estimating what would be the right time to ask her to interrupt the joyful freedom of sliding on ice and stab her fingers in the winter cold, testing her blood sugar levels, as she had done a thousand times before. The blood test results, rather than her own feelings of hunger, would determine whether or not she needed to consume carbohydrates.

Watching Danai´s face made me very happy. It was a face lit with joy; she measured her blood sugar very quickly and ate some carbohydrates even faster, all while standing on the ice—eager to escape from the demands, pain, and obligations of diabetes and get back to the interesting, essential, and happy moment she was living. She wanted to leave behind the painful aspects of her reality as fast as possible and return to the challenge of balancing on ice without falling, because that was why she was here, like so many others around her. This experience filled me with optimism. Once again, I could see diabetes and its demands becoming secondary. Under the influence of pleasant, festive stimuli, Danai was not intimidated—in fact, she was not even thinking about the risk of hypoglycemia. This was one of the first times since leaving the hospital when we all witnessed the positive effect a well-balanced psychological state can have on the body. The levels of sugar in Danai's blood were proof of that.

15. UNLIMITED DEMANDS: DANAI´S PSYCHOLOGICAL WORLD

I will never know how Danai´s personality would have evolved, had she not been diabetic. From a very young age, she demonstrated the ability to adjust very quickly to environmental changes. From the start, she always seemed to enjoy the challenge of new experiences, jumping out of bed at any time of night to race to get ready for another flight to an unknown destination, an unknown world where she would meet people of other ethnicities, sleep in new beds, taste new tastes, and hear and speak other languages, all with a permanent smile on her face. I remember how her smile as a small child reflected her emotional balance and the confidence that she was safe and her life was predictable. Danai's facial expressions and attitude showed that she was happy, wherever and however she lived.

She adjusted fast to school life and to the birth of her sister, despite losing her status as the only child in the family. She never seemed afraid of any situation, even when visiting her pediatrician or another doctor. She appeared to feel safe in her physical integrity, secure and confident in her own ability to accomplish tasks. She adapted to the flow of life naturally, without complications or objections.

From very early on, Danai's sunny disposition was admired and commented on, not only by relatives and friends but also by people who met her in the street—especially old ladies— who were stunned by this little girl's enthusiasm, joy, and the inner peace she exuded while discovering her world. When we stopped by a garden with beautifully fragrant roses, I used to lift her up and let her stick her nose into one, to smell its beautiful aroma. She expressed joy and a sense of inner peace every time she picked up soil, stones, or twigs in her hands and whenever she threw a banana skin into a brook and followed its course. Danai loved to pick up a snail and watch it retreat inside its shell. She did her best to fly up to the sky in a swing, happy that she was getting so close to the clouds. When she was three years old, this little girl, permanently alert, raced around quickly on her red bike. I was constantly with her, witnessing the energy that emanated from her young body; it captivated me, filling me with enormous joy and tranquility. Until diabetes arrived.

The demands of type one diabetes are permanent; the diabetic child cannot escape them. This permanence has an impact on the mind as well as the body. It crushes any attempt to free yourself from its net, imposing oppressive feelings and forcing the diabetic person onto a roller coaster of psychological states. Diabetes makes people feel they have reached a dead end many times over.

Type one diabetics shoulder the responsibility for regulating the functions of their bodies, knowing that a mistake or miscalculation could have serious and unpleasant consequences. I will never know how Danai would have evolved psychologically had she not been diabetic, but I have serious reasons to suspect that diabetes played and continues to play a significant role in the formation of her personality. I understand her multiple, self-evident reasons for feeling betrayed, disappointed, sad, and desperate. Her desire to end the constant effort to keep body and mind in balance is understandable and legitimate. I see how much more saturated and psychologically drained she can be than a non-diabetic child.

My diabetic child seems prone to a wide range of mood swings, positive and negative, experienced with a different intensity every time. I often interpret Danai´s changing reactions as a natural consequence of everything she has to endure: the low and high levels of sugar in her blood, the headaches and the fatigue when hyperglycemic, the vision problems, the rapid heartbeat, weakness and trembling when hypoglycemic, the thousands of punctures in her fingers and body, the hurtful and inconsiderate comments of other children, the loss of the freedom and carefree living she only managed to get a taste of during the first eight years of her life, the school excursions she missed because of her special needs, the permanent feeling of being different, her inability to decide when, how much, and which food to consume, the interruptions to everyday life, the sleeping disorders, and the joys of life sacrificed on the altar of diabetes—to list only a few.

The serious responsibility this eight-year-old girl was forced to shoulder so abruptly put the brakes on childlike spontaneity. It mangled her smile and replaced it with sorrow. Diabetes interrupted her innocence, joy, and carefree life in a violent and harsh way. What really made me worry was that this condition started to impede Danai's willingness to test her own abilities and spread her wings toward independence. Diabetes made her overly reliant on her parents, slowing down an essential process of psychological development. It impeded her natural ability to learn to survive without us supervising and continuously coordinating her movements. Under these circumstances, there was an obvious risk that Danai would develop a faulty impression of herself as helpless, vulnerable, and unable to function without help from other people. None of these feelings were—or should have been—part of the natural development of a child of her age; they were unenviable and unwelcome.

16. ANTIDOTES AGAINST PAIN

No living organism can endure for a prolonged period of time the strain of negative emotions without collapsing. Constantly having to tolerate type one diabetes is an enormous task which leaves scars. From her diagnosis to the present, Danai has often reached saturation point—feeling helpless and unable to fight. Several times, her psyche seemed to lose its wings and fall. When that happened, I had to grab it by the hand and pull it back up to where it belonged. At moments like these, I always had an ace up my sleeve to use as an antidote to pain: the golden prescription the diabetologist gave me, a few hours before we left the hospital. I let this prescription function as my magic filter many times; it was my source of strength when I had to give strength. "You should not let diabetes dominate your lives," the doctor advised me at the start of our struggle. I followed her advice as well as I could, wherever I could.

One of the things I have learned in life is that humans are especially receptive to positive messages and open to advice when facing demanding situations. It is best to reward a person first with praise. When giving advice, it is more efficient to start by acknowledging the degree of difficulty a person is facing and to demonstrate compassion for the pain he or she is in. Danai is no exception to that rule. Occasionally, I let her know that I am aware of how much she struggles with diabetes. I praise her for coping with the demands of her condition as best she can.

During critical moments, when Danai is overwhelmed by negative emotions, one strategy I apply to alleviate frustration is to remind her that life is so much more than meets the eye. I tell her that there are many things to enjoy, not just needles, pain and measurements. It is up to her to choose to engage and fill up her life with pleasant activities. At difficult moments, when Danai has reached the point of saturation and despair, I sometimes ask her to do a simple calculation. If one day consists of 24 hours, then she needs around two of those hours to manage her diabetes. I remind her that she therefore has 22 hours left, and is free to decide how she wants to spend them. It is up to her to decide how to use those hours, without letting diabetes overshadow her ideas for a creative, active and joyful life. In this way, she can give herself an opportunity to learn and develop.

Living with my diabetic child, I have come to believe that, compared with non-diabetic children Danai has a greater need to feel almost constantly able to take the initiative in forming her own world the way she wants to. The realization: "I can decide for myself how I am going to spend my time and my life" offers fertile ground for optimism; it frees the soul, offering a fresh start to every hour, every day, and every month in a life with diabetes. Beyond school obligations and the time she has to spend managing her condition, it is important for Danai's mental balance that she is offered ample opportunities to decide how she wants to spend her free time and can put these decisions into practice. This way, she gets the chance to fill up the sack of her own life experiences with precious smaller and larger treasures, with new impressions and sounds, and with new colors and tastes that she has chosen for herself.

During especially difficult moments, I try not to let Danai become drawn too deeply into the swirl of demands and restrictions that accompany diabetes. I remind her not to forget to live here and now as best she can. At moments like these, I try to encourage her to enjoy the small and greater joys of life. I am convinced that it's essential for her not to get lost in oceans of sorrow, but to look for small and precious harbors of happiness. In this way, I hope that someday, when a solution to the riddle of type one diabetes is found, her sack of life experiences will be filled with worthy, beautiful, favorite, loving, and creative memories too heavy to lift, while the little bag carrying the demands of diabetes will have become an important life lesson. Over time, as we took small steps along the path of our new life, we had to learn to give diabetes a secondary status. This is the attitude I wanted Danai to adopt, especially during moments of despair. Her smiling face and willingness to engage in many different activities made me hope that I was managing to achieve exactly that.

Among the many challenges a diabetic child is called to face is the painful realization that diabetes may be a permanent condition (at least given what we currently know). I believe that diabetic children extract a lot of healing, not only through feeling free to decide how to plan their own lives, but also through the conviction that their condition is only permanent for now. As an additional antidote to pain, I therefore remind Danai that nothing is permanent, especially in the area of diabetes research and therapies. I want her to hope, as I do, that the efforts of many scientists around the world, all working hard to understand this condition, will be fruitful and that these scientists will find a solution to this riddle. I remind Danai that until this happens, we have to use the methods of treating diabetes that are available to us today to help make her life easier.

At moments of crisis, I have called on extraordinary people and their ways of life. Another antidote to pain that has proved especially helpful during times of unbearable pressure for Danai (and equally useful for liberating mind and psyche) is focusing on examples of other diabetic people and their accomplishments. Despite the need to schedule their lives, these people nevertheless show an even greater determination and willingness to experience adventures. These daring individuals show us how many different life scenarios diabetics can participate in, even under the shadow of their condition and its demands, provided that they do not allow diabetes to dominate their lives.

One such valuable lesson was the beautiful example of a thirty-year-old type one diabetic woman who spoke at a conference in Germany. She showed us the schedule she followed when she decided to take part in a triathlon. Her personal account taught us how a diabetic athlete could survive a grueling competition. She told us how she kept glucose in her sleeves while swimming. She couldn't swim with her insulin pump, but volunteers made sure that it was ready to use and waiting with her bicycle when she came out. She explained how, even while cycling, she managed to measure her blood sugar and consume carbohydrates stored in special bags. This woman's performance was amazing; she came sixth in the competition. It was even more amazing to hear, through her personal story, about someone who was living proof that whoever lives his or her life with passion and love, stamina and confidence forces the power of diabetes to fade away, giving this special condition a lessened status.

This athlete's personal account made me feel more human, especially when I heard how many people stood by her side during every minute of her achievement. Doctors, trainers, and volunteers helped her schedule her training and closely supervised her performance, adjusting the amount of insulin she was taking to the needs of each activity, while encouraging her with obvious enthusiasm and contributing to the achievement of her goal. I stored in my memory forever the ruddy cheeks, well-trained body, and sparkling eyes of this vibrant figure—a diabetic athlete filled with life energy, even as she was presenting to us a detailed analysis of her blood sugar fluctuations during a training session. In her, I saw someone who did not let diabetes become an obstacle in her life or interfere with her right to have dreams and ambitions about her future and to accomplish them. As soon as I got home, I described the experience to Danai with great joy, handing over to her another precious piece for her own puzzle.

There are many examples of people who have chosen to go on enjoying the privilege of being alive, while accepting the fact that they are in one way different from others. I think of the precious lessons our family learned about stamina and strength of character when we were lucky enough to be present at the Paralympic Games, those amazing moments we experienced in Athens in 2004. I did not know then that what Danai and I witnessed inside the Olympic Stadium would become a source of optimism for both of us many years later. We saw the impressive determination of athletes competing in their chosen sports, athletes who were different from the norm because they had lost one or more limbs. I wanted my children, despite their young age, to become familiar with the accomplishments of people with different abilities and the challenges they faced. It was a good opportunity to learn that the ones among us with special needs deserve as much respect as the rest of the population.

Danai was just four years old at that event. However, what she experienced was so life-changing that she still remembers very clearly not only the Olympic flame we were privileged to be close to, but also the athletes competing in their chosen sports, using bodies that were not intact. We have discussed these special human beings on a number of occasions since then, whenever Danai seemed to have reached another dead end and needed special treatment to achieve a moral uplift. The echo of their accomplishments and the messages they communicated still support us, despite the passing of so many years.

Other allies in my attempts to boost Danai´s weakened morale have included a group of Chinese monks, the Shaolin, who are athletes with extraordinary skills. The Shaolin monks subject themselves to a number of painful physical trials to train and strengthen not only their bodies but also (and mainly) their minds. Danai knows about and admires the Shaolin. Their philosophy and approach have helped me support her at times of hopelessness or crisis, when she seemed overwhelmed by her physical and mental pain. The Shaolin are another ace to pull out of my sleeve under difficult circumstances, when Danai's tenacity is weakening before the demands of diabetes.

At such moments, I would ask the Shaolin to come and help, to "take" Danai into their team because she too is a kind of fighter. I would ask them to help her bear whatever her condition was forcing her to bear. The parallel, whenever I jokingly explained that she too was a Shaolin fighter, worked wonders. I have the impression that, at such moments, Danai thought about the young men and boys who, despite intense physical pain, balance their bodies on standing swords for an extended period of time. I guessed that she was visualizing the young monks hitting sacks of rice with their fingers thousands of times a day, despite the pain, or jumping into the air and doing acrobatics. At moments like these, Danai seemed to realize how much physical pain those young men were willing to endure in order to raise their minds a step higher.

Whenever I called Danai a "Shaolin fighter," she gave me the impression that she too was willing to endure physical pain, as those Chinese monks do. Whatever her actual mental process, it was clear that she relaxed and derived strength from the wisdom of this ancient martial art, realizing that our tolerance of physical pain is much greater than we believe it to be. Once more, I witnessed the impact that our minds have on our bodies. This experience showed me how any psychological or physical discomfort depends on our state of mind. It allowed me to remind Danai that it is up to us to decide how to use our mental power to get rid of anything that torments us. Such examples renewed my determination not to let the infinitely small period of time allocated to the care of diabetes demoralize Danai or bring her to another dead end.

I used the example of athletes again when discussing the pain in Danai's fingers, pierced multiple times to measure the level of sugar in her blood. This unpleasant part of her ritual occasionally increased her discomfort. But instead of sharing my own pain and reinforcing her distress, I reminded her of the condition of the fingers and toes of some professional tennis players. Danai and I have both witnessed the pain caused by physical abuse when the seriously injured and bandaged toes of a particular tennis player were exposed to millions of spectators during a broadcast game. Often these players needed medical help in order to finish the game.

This was a good opportunity for me to compare athletic injuries with the damage a needle causes to the fingers of a diabetic measuring his or her blood sugar. The image on the screen undoubtedly proved that people could tolerate excessive amounts of pain when they wanted to reach a target. I am sure that Danai compared the condition of her fingers to the condition of those athletes' toes, a contrast that helped to alleviate her psychic pain, while at the same time increasing her inner strength and tolerance.

17. LITTLE CONCOCTIONS, IDEAS, AND TRICKS FOR A LIFE WITH PECULIARITIES

Diabetes is a permanent member of our family. I have accepted it as a special condition of the body and not as a disease. I refuse to consider my child a sick person. To me, sick people are unable to fulfill their duties. The sick have to give up their activities, stay in bed, and take medicine until they recover. By contrast, type one diabetics who respect the seriousness of their condition and take the necessary steps to regulate it, can go unnoticed for most of the day, in the same way as someone who suffers from allergies. Without wanting to draw a likeness between these two physical conditions, since diabetes undoubtedly makes more serious demands, I hope that Danai can adopt a positive way of thinking that does not allow her to experience her body as weak or defeated, or to feel permanently diseased.

For the same reason, I believe it is my responsibility to discourage her from ever using diabetes to evoke pity, even unconsciously. By adopting this attitude, I hope to inspire Danai not to engage with life as an unable, ill-fated person, despite holding a serious disability identity card. I feel that she benefits from not being overprotected or permitted to live the life of a vulnerable, unfortunate sufferer. I make sure that Danai participates in routine chores, such as cleaning the house and emptying the dishwasher. I expect her to help care for our pets and to be primarily responsible for keeping her own room tidy.

It is equally important to continue to point out to Danai that she owes it to herself to appreciate opportunities to use her talents and abilities in the best possible way. It is my responsibility to teach my diabetic child to adopt the attitude that, with the right planning, a lot can be achieved, even while living with diabetes. My wish is for Danai to incorporate into her way of thinking the conviction that type one diabetics can run marathons, study, and write music—in short, can live the lives they want to live.

Although our way of life has changed, we have chosen to continue living life to the full. Since our first flight to Athens with diabetes, we have included a number of activities in our lives, such as going on many excursions. Our need to adjust to the demands of diabetes made me invent ways to help Danai overcome practical problems. I bought a pocket flashlight and attached it to her key-ring so that she could measure her blood sugar levels in the darkness of a movie theater while watching a favorite movie, without needing to interrupt a pleasurable activity that can take her away from the troubles of diabetes.

Another pleasurable activity we continued to enjoy after the diagnosis was visiting our favorite Fun Park. There we could feed animals, take train rides, slide on huge slides, and jump on trampolines, even if Danai did have to regularly put on the brakes and measure her blood sugar, drink juice, and consume carbohydrates. I use special moments like these to show her, through hands-on experience, how much she can accomplish and how many beautiful moments her life can hold, despite her special needs. During such moments of excitement, I take the opportunity to remind Danai that we give ourselves more chances to taste life and enjoy new experiences than many who face no physical complications but simply prefer the familiarity of a routine. Despite diabetes, we are more open to new knowledge and adventure than many non-diabetics, who deprive themselves of the joy of learning, achieving, and exploring unknown territories.

Often, during happy and relaxing moments (for example, when Danai was lying on a picnic blanket with her hands under her head, satisfied with the pleasures of the day), I grabbed the opportunity to remind her that we could still do everything we used to do, and that we would go on having a good time despite the changes that accompany life with diabetes. Through new impressions, Danai learned that diabetes would not prevent her from enjoying large and small happy moments, provided that we were willing to search for simple, alternative solutions.

Such realizations have a greater and more uplifting impact on a child's morale when the theory is put into practice. When Danai not only hears that diabetes need not be a burden, but actually experiences that truth, the positive effect on her spirit is striking. Every action or happily lived moment provides tangible proof that most of the restrictions we feel in our lives are caused by our way of thinking—they are obstacles and limits we impose on ourselves.

18. MY FIRST YEAR WITH DIABETES: ISOLATION, DEPRESSION, AND MORE...

The first year with diabetes turned out to be especially difficult and demanding for me, in relation to what followed. While all my energy was invested in meeting new demands and all my senses were directed towards the task of caring for my children, I was also watching my own inner world change. Various symptoms of depression became my new reality. My body was forced into inactivity. I could not and did not want to organize any outings or meetings with other people. I needed to be alone with my thoughts, to isolate myself. What could I have done to prevent what my child was now going through? When did her pancreas start not functioning properly? When did her body begin to destroy its own cells? Where was I then and what was I doing? What kind of future was my child going to have? Diabetes was an accomplished fact; my own weakness and inability to prevent or reverse its permanence were tearing me to pieces.

During the first year of Danai's diagnosis, my mind often oscillated like a pendulum between the past and the present. I lived as if my feet were planted on two different pieces of ice: one in the past, in the era before diabetes, and the other in the present, in a very different reality that I did not want to accept. I felt as if the two pieces were floating in icy water and drifting apart, according to their own rules, indifferent to my own need to survive.

The tendency I had, during that period, to constantly compare the past with the present, the times before and after diabetes, caused a succession of mainly negative feelings. I automatically compared every situation I found myself in to an equivalent situation in the past. With every step and breath, I thought about how our lives used to be, before our visit to the pediatrician: two weeks, one month, two months ago—what everything was like a year ago when we were celebrating birthdays, and at Christmas, Easter, and during the summer vacation. I remembered how Danai used to live without injecting insulin, without hypoglycemia, without suffering, fear, or sadness. All of this existed and was so wonderful in the past! I clung to the deep satisfaction I remembered experiencing during our carefree early years. I tortured myself with calculations, additions, and subtractions, with the before and after and the threatening permanence of the new.

Memories suddenly recurred with an intensity that was mentally crippling. The present hurt so much that I would have done anything to avoid it. Perhaps the unbearable pain of the present and my unwillingness to accept our new reality caused me to search for refuge in the past. I needed to feel, even for a short time, a feeling of warmth and joy that the present could not provide; for that reason, I refused to let go of the past. I co-opted whatever I could to remain mentally in the pre-diabetes era. I used the papers piled up on my desk, leaving them untouched for a long time. I decided not to return to my usual sports center, because I trained there before diabetes came to torment Danai. I was afraid to go back to the old places, because I knew they would force me to make the before and after comparison.

At the same time, I felt frozen in the realization that what I was looking for did not exist and would never exist again.

The psychological pressure was enormous and long lasting. As a result, I no longer functioned as well as before. On one occasion, I experienced a feeling so intense and peculiar that it made me realize how much strain I was actually under. It made me think that what I was going through—an unprocessed psychological stage—was threatening my mental balance. I came face to face with a new dimension of myself. It happened one day when I was shopping at a supermarket. I suddenly felt that my body and mind were unable to function. It took me only a few seconds to realize that I did not have enough energy left to set myself in motion. I could not continue to think. I did not want to make any more decisions about banal questions—such as which of the multitude of products in this shop we needed at home. Suddenly, I was trapped in a huge contradiction: I was unable to move and, at the same time, felt an intense urge to abandon the place I was in as fast as possible. I felt I had reached a real dead end, with my soul trapped inside my body.

With great difficulty and under enormous pressure, I managed to stop shopping and drive home. I climbed the stairs up to our flat without wanting to get there, perhaps because our living space was loaded with tensions and responsibilities I did not want to shoulder, or perhaps because it was full of pictures I did not want to store in my memory. As I had no other choice, I went in and sat down. I did not have the stamina to do anything more. I sank onto the sofa and became immersed in an immeasurable psychological vacuum, a sensation I often experienced during the period that followed.

When I found myself suspended in this vacuum, I made a decision. I had to isolate myself. I would make whatever effort was needed to carry out the tasks in my routine; I was willing to be there for my children and their needs. I did not need the company of others and I did not want to explain how I was feeling or living. I did not want to see faces full of pity or experience people's superficial interest in social surroundings. I did not want to have to satisfy anyone's curiosity. I did not want people unable to feel what it meant for an eight-year-old child to live with diabetes to drain away my precious energy (or what was left of it). I did not want to share my time with people who were mere observers, demanding that I pay attention to their own self-centered, meaningless desires. I did not see why I should give in to the pressure to put sentiment behind me and quickly start functioning the way I had before Danai's diagnosis.

In fact, my life as the mother of a child with type one diabetes was an individual and lonely path that I had to follow to the end. I did not want other people telling me to distance myself as fast as possible from painful negative feelings, because I wanted to let those feelings do their natural work. I respected their existence and paid attention to them. Negative feelings carry important and precious messages; they can become genuine teachers if we attend to them at the appropriate time and listen carefully to what they are telling us. I wanted to live through this experience fully, letting it take its natural course.

Isolation was what I needed and sought. Without isolating myself, I knew I could not put things in order. During those very first moments with diabetes, I needed to experience uncomfortable feelings. They made me feel real, and were appropriate to the circumstances. My emotional world was the natural outcome of what had happened some days earlier. There was no reason to turn a blind eye, pretend I had everything under control, or present a false face and refuse to admit that I was living with symptoms of depression.

I accepted my depression. I looked it straight in the eye and it looked back at me. We kept each other company. I reconciled myself and it allowed me to learn. Wasn't this the right time to feel depressed? Why show a happy face when I wasn't happy? There was no reason to be dishonest with myself. I did not want to have to defend my emotional world. I did not want to be fake. If I had any freedom left to make choices, then it should be possible to choose to be authentic. I really needed to retreat to allow body and mind to experience what they needed to experience. Otherwise, I would not be respecting my own vital need to have some respite, break away, reshuffle ideas, revise thoughts, look for solutions, and regenerate.

I was in a new and unpleasant reality, but it was my reality and I had to accept it. Depression, I had always believed, is a natural outcome when a person experiences loss: the loss of a good job, a good friendship, one's own country, a loved one, dignity, health, one's own home, the freedom of expression, physical and mental freedom, or the privilege of becoming a parent. Moreover, loss is a basic condition that forces you to abandon the throne you were sitting on before the change. It makes you leave the warmth, affection, predictability, and comfort of the familiar. A loss pushes you out of the space where you believed you functioned well. It shakes you violently and forces you into the new and unknown, which can be awkward and frightening. It takes you to a place where you have to contrive new ways to survive and open new paths to walk down.

Not only through my profession, but also through private interactions, I have become familiar with many different personal stories. I have observed a pattern of behavior common to many: how the pain and untreated wounds we carry for lifetimes can limit our spiritual evolution. I have come to acknowledge the therapeutic quality of accepting and consciously experiencing negative emotions, such as sorrow, desperation, the feeling of emptiness, insecurity, fear, and the feeling of being unable to function as well as before. I believe this to be an integral part of the reality we call life. The conscious experiencing of negative emotions is the healthy reaction of an organism responding to a traumatic event.

Back then, when the influence of Danai's diagnosis was exercising absolute control over my emotional life, I felt that accepting the energy of the unpleasant and allowing myself to consciously experience its full power—making no effort to delude myself or compromise— would enable me to receive some benefit. It was the only way to turn this painful phase of my life into an emotional cure. I was not willing to waste this learning opportunity, simply for the sake of presenting a fake but agreeable picture of myself to others.

Back then, when depression was my permanent companion, I thought of feelings, positive and negative, as clothes for the soul. Each piece hangs on the line; each one has a function. They are all waiting for the soul to come and decide what to wear. Who would want to be responsible for taking or keeping any of those options off the line? Which clothes aren't needed? Who wants to decide which feelings should be allowed on the washing line?

In my isolation, I felt that by denying the existence of the unpleasant, I would automatically be denying the existence of the pleasant. If I did not allow myself to live in darkness, how could I appreciate light? If I did not accept sorrow, I would never appreciate happiness, prosperity, or satisfaction. Denying this anguish would impose a cruel order on my psyche and mangle it painfully—like forcing a wounded horse to run a race.

Recently, a doctor specializing in acupuncture told me about the amazing ability of the human body to judge for itself how long and in which places to hold onto acupuncture needles, waiting until all their benefits are acquired before letting them fall. I liked what that doctor said. It was one more example of the wisdom of nature, which the human organism is part of. I believe that feelings have a similar function in the psyche to acupuncture needles in the body. Whether positive or negative, they appear and disappear repetitively, they circulate like sea waves, arriving one after another. During my depression, I felt I had to let negative feelings do their job before positive ones could come to the surface and replace them. Given that it was the right time for negative feelings to be active, I wanted to experience all their tension until my system did not need them anymore, and could reject them. To force myself in another direction was the last thing I needed. My instinct pointed me toward isolation as an emergency solution and an opportunity for reorientation, self-observation, and analysis of the situation I was in. I trust the wisdom of human nature, and was not willing to ignore the messages I was receiving.

This period was a time to work on accepting the new reality. I sought isolation partly because it was all I could bear, and partly because I needed it to create the conditions for a positive outcome. My mental state made me slow down the rhythm of my fast-paced life and gave me an opportunity to analyze what the diagnosis of diabetes really meant for us. Amidst the isolation I had consciously chosen, inside the fortress I had built around myself, my physical activity slowed down but my mental activity was increasing. During the first days, weeks, and months after the diagnosis, others probably thought I was idle, but I knew that I was very busy with my inner world. I was starting to realize that I had to become very cautious about what benefited or harmed me, and constantly on the alert for ways to help my children. I was not willing to compromise on that.

In the long run, accepting my negative emotions and consciously experiencing them weakened my pain and established a new balance. In time, the iceberg of the past on which I was still standing with one leg began to melt, decrease in size, and lose its power; at the same time, the piece of ice beneath my other leg, representing the present, seemed to gain substance and size. That world began to dominate and press for acceptance. I realized that I had to decide whether there was any benefit in attempting to stand on something that had no substance anymore, the world before diabetes, which I desperately clung to. It was up to me to decide whether and for how long I would expose my inner balance to danger. It was for me to choose whether to continue clinging to the past, which would never return, or to plant both legs in the present. My internal Darwinian mechanism for adjusting to new demands did not seem to function instantly or with complete effectiveness. I knew that, like the butterflies in Manchester, I needed time to say farewell to my colorful wings and learn to survive under different circumstances.

19. DANAI AND ME: SIGNS OF RECOVERY

The first weeks after the diagnosis, or rather the first months, I could see that Danai was intensively occupied, not only with the reactions of her body, but also with what was going on beyond and around her. She gave me the impression of needing to feel that at least some things had gone back to normal. I felt that she wanted to live as much as possible in the same way as before, as if familiar conditions could somehow preserve her inner balance and foster her development. I could see that my child, especially then, needed both her relationship with me and my everyday behavior to stay the same. She wanted to see me continuing to do everything I did before our stay in the hospital. Before her diagnosis, I used to sit and study for hours on end for my university final exams. I used to go to the university and out for other engagements, and I used to answer all my emails.

For a long time after our return from the hospital, I never even approached my desk or attempted to return to my normal routine. Danai frequently asked when I would start studying again for the university exams. She wanted to know why I had stopped meeting people at the university and taking steps towards accomplishing my goals. I avoided giving her an honest answer. I did not want her to know what I was feeling, that my future was now determined by diabetes. Danai observed me and I observed her. We were observing each other out of love and concern for each other's wellbeing.

At some point, months after we left the hospital, something happened that forced me to abandon the position I had pinned myself down in. Two events took place that fit together as well as a key fits its lock, and they unlocked my soul. The first was what I saw in my rear-view mirror, while putting the car in reverse for a drive with the kids. Danai was sitting in the back seat, in her usual thoughtful mood, observing me and probably comparing our lives to what they had been in the past and would be in the future. During such periods of contemplation, she often came up with questions. Before I had changed feet on the pedals to drive forward, she asked an unexpected question: when I was planning to go back to university again? I suppose she wanted to know when her life would return to the familiar rhythms she remembered. I knew that I had neither the stamina nor the courage to fulfill her wishes.

I immediately told her the truth, that I had decided to interrupt my studies in order to have more time with my children. The silence in the back seat made me look in the mirror, and what I saw made me turn around at once. The sorrow overflowing in Danai's face terrified me. I had never seen so much sadness in that face before, not even at the hospital, when I explained her diagnosis. I froze. While we drove toward the dance school, I began to wonder whether I had made the right decision about my future.

"No," my husband sounded a note of warning when I told him, some hours later, what had happened in the car. His comment was the second event, which also helped to unlock my soul. He was of the opinion that when Danai realized, sometime in the future, that I had given up all of my personal ambitions because of her diabetes, it would put her under much more strain than the diabetes itself. I thought about what he said over and over again and I did not like the way it made me feel. I did not want to cause Danai any more distress than she already felt. I was there to help her and not to cause additional problems.

I accepted my husband's comment as a warning, alerting me to a problem that I had to find an immediate solution for. This, together with Danai's sad expression, became the driving force that dragged me out of the state I'd been in since the hospital. Maternal love showed me the road I had to follow to start living more and more in the present. Messages of self-preservation stormed my consciousness, warning me about the risks of depriving myself of a creative life, or what I considered to be one. How useful could chronic depression really be? I began to realize that I had to build my reality from scratch—to pick up my pieces and move on. I reminded myself that life gives us endless opportunities to evolve spiritually; I must not miss this opportunity. What was I learning from what I was going through? What would I want my children to learn?

After this incident, I became aware of the fact that I was a role model for my children. I needed to show to them that life goes on, even when it slaps you in the face and you constantly feel the pain of that slap to a greater or a lesser extent. This is true no matter what you do or where you are. What was I planning to do with my time? How could I help Danai avoid becoming entrapped in the demands of diabetes and encourage her to think of herself as someone who was not disabled?

How could I fail to show my child, through my own behavior, how strong I was and how many things we could accomplish, even with diabetes in our lives? Wasn't I the one who had confidently declared, over lunch during our first visit home from the hospital, that diabetes had invaded her life to show her how strong she was? How strong had my own behavior seemed up to that point? How could I fail to practice what I was preaching? What did I want Danai to think of me? What sort of childhood memories would stay with her in adult life, after experiencing diabetes? Did I want my child to remember me as a depressed mother who gave up on life? Did I want her to remember me asking her to be strong when I was weak myself?

My daughter was diagnosed with type one diabetes. In Germany, there are two thousand new cases per year, although no one definitely knows the cause. The nature of this condition is unpredictable and permanent; it would always be part of our lives. I had to accept the unavoidable, sudden turn my child's life had taken, no matter how painful it was. The absolute present is what is tangible, what is real. Whether pleasant or unpleasant, it is our constant companion. What we experience now is powerful, filled with vital energy and substance. My present is a tough reality. It was essential for me to recover morally and psychologically, not only for my own benefit, but also for that of the people I was responsible for. Once again, I had to fall back on the doctor's advice, and refuse to let diabetes dominate my life.

Danai's reaction in the car made me realize, that I urgently needed to evaluate my own attitude and find ways to move on and overcome my sense of resignation. It made me realize that I must not miss out on the present, on life with my children, or on life in general. I began to make an effort to find a way out of this dead end. I chose a path that would lead me toward the creative but difficult, and demanding outside world, hand in hand with our new reality. That was the moment when I began to accept that my child was diabetic and I could not change that fact. Through my own attitude towards diabetes, I would have to support her by wiping the sorrow from her face and giving her the strength to move on with her life. After this intense lesson in the car on the way to the dancing school, I began reconciling myself with the need to become active enough to recreate the rhythms of our past life.

In time, I managed to reach a point where I could think clearly and appreciate the benefits of pursuing my own personal interests. I began to offer myself opportunities to learn and be active, combined with moments of relaxation that helped me cope with the biggest challenge of my life. I arranged to complete my university studies; this turned out to be a much-needed break from the demands of family life. Focusing on an intellectual topic took my mind off depressing realities and was a welcome change. Only then did I realize how quickly everyone else in our family had returned to what they were doing before diabetes entered our lives. Danai went back to school, Ioli continued to go to kindergarten, and my husband went to work.

This was also the time when I received a beautiful gift from my family, a trip abroad to my beloved London. I accepted the gift with great reluctance and only after my family had made multiple, persistent efforts to convince me to go. This trip gave me the chance to spend a long weekend alone, without family obligations, taking part in activities I was interested in. I had doubts about whether I should go so far away from my family. Before the trip, I could not imagine how beneficial it would be, not only for me, but also for Danai. The three days I spent in London taught both of us a valuable lesson: when the person who usually cares for you leaves for a short time, it means that you are well and your existence is not under threat, because otherwise this person you trust would not leave you. When you take time away from the people you care for every day, you acknowledge their right to learn to survive without being absolutely and constantly dependent on you. You acknowledge their right and obligation to learn to paddle their own canoes.

The three-day trip to London did more than help me relax and recover; it also made me realize, once again, that our children are not our property. Parents are, or should be, fellow travelers on their children's path of life. We should stay beside them to guide them as best we can, encouraging them to follow their instincts, make use of their talents, and accomplish their goals. This three-day trip made me appreciate that the job of parents is to provide their children with the support they need to fulfill ambitions that will give them a sense of satisfaction. We should be there as guides, while at the same time letting them decide what to do in their lives. We should offer our children, and especially the ones with special needs, the opportunity to exist as unique individuals, learning to survive without our constant presence.

20. WORKING TOWARD A GOOD SYMBIOSIS WITH DIABETES

Although I managed to change the attitude I had adopted during my period of isolation, the issue of diabetes continued to preoccupy me. I began to search intensively for ways to regulate it, reading anything I could lay my hands on about the best nutrition for diabetics. I studied special diets meant to regulate diabetes, which unfortunately proved to be unsuitable for type one diabetics. For quite some time, I adopted the protocol of jotting down exactly what Danai had eaten every day, in relation to the levels of sugar she was measuring in her blood, hoping to draw some conclusions about which foods helped balance those levels and which ones disrupted them.

For a considerable amount of time, diabetes was "talking" to me but I was not listening. It was telling me that it had its own rules and norms. Several times, I thought I had reached my target, only to realize that nutrition was not the only factor affecting Danai's body or creating desirable results. I began to notice that, her blood sugar measurements were the result of a combination of mental, psychological, and physical factors. I began to accept the fact that diabetes is like a wild beast in the jungle, running and playing hide-and-seek with those around it. There is no button you can push to achieve a constant, perfect balance in the diabetic body. Through my observations, I learned that diabetes adopts side partners, including stress, physical activity, happiness and sorrow, the injected insulin, and the body's hormonal fluctuations. I also learned to accept that even when I believed I had done everything right, there was always room for mistakes. The sooner I accepted this fact, the easier our symbiosis with the wild beast would be. In time, after many efforts to tame the peculiar condition affecting my child's body—and after a frenetic search for substances (such as cinnamon) that were supposed to decrease this and increase the other—I stopped searching.

21. ALLIES IN OUR SYMBIOSIS WITH DIABETES: THE FIRST PETS

A few months after Danai was diagnosed with diabetes, we had an experience that demonstrated to us the decisive impact that a state of the mind can have on the body—we got our first pets. Before our odyssey with diabetes began, Danai and Ioli had tried several times to convince me to let them have a pet. There were a number of reasons why I opposed my children's sweet request, and they included my own respect and love for animals. I did not want to force weak-willed creatures to live in unfavorable conditions. I always felt badly about confining an animal to a very restricted space. I also worried that our lack of time and occasional travels would make it hard to have any kind of pet, whether it was a dog, cat, bird, mouse, or fish—anything alive and moving. Both children knew that there was no point lobbying my husband, as I was mainly responsible for managing our daily routine.

When diabetes entered our lives, the children did not stop asking for a pet; instead, the issue became even more pressing. Just weeks after the shock of the hospital, Danai and Ioli renewed their lobbying, hoping to get any sort of creature—preferably hairy—to live with us. When their arguments and requests failed, they decided to try a different approach. On every door in our apartment, they put up big pieces of paper that said, in three languages: "We want rabbits!"

At first, I just laughed at how inventive my children had been, ignoring the essence of their request. I passed the pieces of paper every time I went from one room to the next, hearing them flutter as my movements caused a breeze. "OK kids," I thought, "that's a nice trick to try and change my mind but it won't work!" I didn't want animal hair all over the place, and I didn't want scratched furniture. Most of all, I did not want to be responsible for more lives. Not to talk about the expense! I never doubted the therapeutic effect that animals can have on humans.

I grew up with pets and knew how precious their presence was in my life, but as an adult, I was not ready to take on more responsibilities.

I can't say with certainty how long those posters hung on the doors, or how many times I looked at them, expecting them to disappear just as they had appeared. We went on like this until something happened that shook me and made me change my mind in seconds. Once again, Danai was trying to convince me to buy rabbits. Her basic argument was that our neighbors, two floors below us, who lived in an apartment half the size of ours, with a balcony much smaller than our veranda, had rabbits!

"Why does everything have to be perfect in our life?" she asked, with desperation in her eyes. The child's wisdom had surfaced once again. I knew I had to listen with the respect it deserved. This question echoed through my mind and had a great effect on me. It pinned me down and made me engage in serious thinking. Why does everything in our life have to be perfect? Our life had never been perfect, especially after we began to live with diabetes. If my daughter was forced to accept her condition with a pancreas that wasn't functioning perfectly, if she had to tolerate the pain this imperfection caused, then there was no reason why four-legged creatures couldn't live with us and share these imperfect conditions. These thoughts and realizations crossed my mind in seconds, if in a less detailed and ordered way. I suddenly thought that I had been wrong.

How could I refuse my children´s wish to have some four-legged supporters in their struggle—especially Danai? As their role model, I had an opportunity to demonstrate how a person should adjust to change and try to find solutions to new challenges that arose. Danai gave me a precious lesson through her love of animals. Life does not have to be perfect for us to live it. Some seconds later, she saw that I was transforming and promising to seriously consider their wish. She did not know that I had already decided to find the pets that would, only days later, become members of our family.

Everything happened very fast. As Coello reminds us, the universe conspires; soon after my discussion with Danai, we found ourselves in a stable with many rabbits. The lady who cared for them allowed the children to choose two of the five newly-born hairy little bundles. We would have to wait until the newborns stopped nursing before we could take them home. For the sake of those babies, the children learned to manage the psychological tribulation of waiting. During the period that followed, we were busy organizing the space where our new companions would live. We bought them a house, food, and plates, and bought ourselves a book on how to take care of rabbits. Then we waited for the phone call that would tell us they were ready.

I can still hear the children's cheering and rejoicing when the owner of the rabbits called to say it was time: we could take the babies home and start living with them. At that moment, the needles, pain, fear, agony, sadness, disappointments, hypoglycemia, and all the other trappings of diabetes lost significance. The day we picked up the rabbits, nothing else mattered to Danai and loli apart from those two beings. The measurements, injections, and weighing of food were done very fast without inhibitions or much thought. The unpleasantness of having to manage diabetes faded away amidst intense joy at the prospect of having animals as life partners. Danai had no time or interest to spend thinking about the peculiarities of her condition. That just wasn't important. By getting pets, we were demonstrating our willingness to begin welcoming moments of joy into our lives. Life had slapped us in the face; that didn't mean we had to turn the other cheek.

The two furry siblings, Jeans and Polly, received enormous love and attention from the very beginning. The children's overflowing joy pushed away the sorrow in our house. At Danai's next hospital checkup, the doctor asked: "What happened here?" pointing to the sugar level values we had jotted down in her diabetes diary during the week when the rabbits came home. The doctor wanted to know what had caused the remarkable balance in Danai's physical functions, as shown by her blood sugar levels.

"We bought rabbits," she answered, her eyes sparkling with joy. She seemed to feel that she now had the best allies in the world in her daily battle with diabetes. Perhaps my eyes sparkled with joy too. I wanted to believe that the animals would have a permanent effect on Danai's diabetes. However, the intensive feelings of our first days with the rabbits did not last forever. The initial enthusiasm their arrival caused decreased in intensity; as a result, their positive effect on Danai's blood sugar measurements diminished. In time, the ecstasy of our first days with pets gave way to ordinary happiness, until Jeans and Polly were taken for granted, although they remained a source of love and tranquility. Danai's week of remarkably good blood sugar levels was a wonderful parenthesis in the harsh reality of diabetes. After that period, we went back to the familiar vicissitudes. I had to accept the fact that I could not constantly provide my child with opportunities to reduce the effect of diabetes on her body.

Although we never again experienced such a remarkable and long-lasting balancing of Danai's diabetes, even four years later, when two more pets (the tomcats, Heraklis and Dias) joined the family, we never stopped trying to fill our lives with beautiful moments. Compared to the pre-diabetes era, we had fewer activities, but the ones that remained helped us discover lost parts of ourselves. We did not feel defeated. We had to look for new ways to survive and feel that we still existed and could somehow function. We needed to feel that we had not lost everything, even though the carpet had been suddenly pulled out from under our feet. The effort to adjust to our new lives would have made Darwin happy: at least one group of people was trying to put his theory into practice.

22. ONE MORE CHALLENGE TO FACE: CELIAC DISEASE

After living with diabetes for a year, I had to emerge from deep despair and negative emotions to accept its terms and conditions. Danai, although not indifferent to the fact that she was diabetic, seemed more and more to be coming to terms with the idea that she would have to live with this peculiar condition. We had learned our lessons; we had been brave and strong; we had demonstrated many times a willingness to go on. And then, one day at lunch, when we were committed to not giving up and tasting the joys life offered, the phone rang.

Who would disturb us at this time of day? People who knew us well understood that lunch was a critical time, when Danai injected insulin and ate. The meal always had to be ready at a precise time because she might come home from school hypoglycemic. Family and friends refrained from calling during lunch, so I was absolutely certain that whoever was calling had nothing to do with the world of diabetes. I picked up the phone. I was wrong. The voice of Danai's diabetologist greeted me cheerfully. He wanted to know what we were up to. I told him that Danai had just had her insulin, hoping he would realize that the next few minutes were crucial. He knew that once the insulin started working in her body, she needed to consume carbohydrates quickly. The last thing I wanted to do just then was talk on the phone.

But the doctor was thrilled with his success at tracing me and wanted to talk about a number of things. As he was my daughter's doctor and not a friend, I could not do what I wanted and let him know it was a bad time. Instead, I let him talk, struggling to be part of the conversation while preparing lunch. Undaunted, he asked me whether we had received a reply to our letter.

That letter—whether we had sent it, resent it, or received some kind of answer—was for a long time one of the diabetologist's main concerns; he mentioned it every time we came to the hospital for Danai´s scheduled check-up. He wanted parents to write to the management of the hospital to express dissatisfaction with how it was operating. He himself was unhappy with the way different sections of his working environment functioned. He used to tell us how many times he got into arguments with people in these sections without achieving what he wished to achieve.

For some reason, the doctor was convinced that parents could make a difference. He therefore constantly reminded us to send letters of complaint. We respected his request and wrote to the hospital management, mentioning the deficiencies we had noticed during our stay. They had to do with the way the hospital functioned, and the mistakes staff members made that were relevant to the treatment of diabetes. We mentioned the impact that the shortage of diabetologists had on us, when we urgently needed the help of a specialist. Most of the time, we sought help over the phone; a number of times we were left alone with our problem. We soon found out that the help we received (if any) depended on the hospital doctors´ shifts. To our dismay, on many nights there was no diabetologist available at the hospital. Instead, staff members had to phone specialists at home for advice. All of these experiences were mentioned in our letter.

We never thought that a written complaint from us would make much of an impact on the way the hospital was run, but we wrote a letter nevertheless. During that lunchtime phone call, I had to disappoint Danai's diabetologist, pointing out that nobody had shown the slightest interest in the mistakes we wrote about, as parents of a diabetic child. I had to tell him that no one had responded, something that was expected and not surprising. Personally, I was worried about issues that meant more to me than whether or not I'd received a reply from the hospital managers. During that phone call, I felt that my daughter's doctor was pursuing utopias, something I could not afford to do.

As I answered the diabetologist's question, I tried to signal that I was running out of time and needed to end our conversation. I felt I was under enormous pressure, still worrying about the effect Danai's insulin was having on her body. It was hard to believe the doctor still had topics to discuss, but he seemed unwilling to put down the receiver, something that made the time pressure feel immense.

It was five days before Danai's twelfth birthday and we had already organized her party. We had ordered a cake and she had invited many of her friends. It was Monday, just like that afternoon four years earlier, when Danai and I had played hangman at the pediatrician's office. On the phone, the otherwise likeable doctor asked whether I remembered the blood test he had carried out, the last time we were in the hospital. Of course I remembered—I was the one who had reminded him to do it. The results of the test were back, he told me, as I stood in the kitchen with the wooden spoon in my hand, watching my children, who were waiting for me to have lunch. The results showed that there was some kind of problem with Danai's small intestine. We would have to make an appointment to admit her to the hospital, where doctors would carry out an endoscopic examination to decide whether the blood test results were valid. Danai would have to stay in the hospital for several days and undergo an examination under full anesthesia. The doctor wished me a pleasant day and said we could talk more about this issue at our next meeting, which would take place soon. Then he hung up and let me carry on with my daily routine.

How I wished I could drop the receiver and pretend our conversation hadn't happened. How I wished we had finished the call after talking about the hospital managers not responding to our letter. How I wished our discussion had ended there, and I could just organize the food, serve my children, have lunch with them, and talk about school. Once more, things did not turn out the way I wanted. Once more, I started to go through the familiar process of denying what was overwhelming me. I could not afford to have a detailed discussion with the diabetologist in front of the children, who were listening to our conversation. I had to set this problem aside and pretend that the doctor had only called to find out about the letter, which was important to him and needed to be dealt with. One reason why I did not want the children to find out immediately was that it wouldn´t be right to spoil Danai´s birthday party. I did not want to spoil the joy of receiving gifts, her happy moments laughing with friends, having fun, eating birthday cake, and enjoying the activities planned for her twelfth birthday. As it would take some time to make an appointment for the medical examinations the doctor had told me about, we could wait until the party was over.

Some days later, before Danai´s birthday, I had another conversation with the same doctor. This time I was home alone and could talk freely. I wanted to know exactly what the blood test results showed. Danai was suffering from celiac disease. Twenty percent of type one diabetic children are affected by celiac disease, he told me, perhaps hoping to boost my morale, something he did not achieve. Danai´s organism could not tolerate cereals such as wheat, rye, oats, or barley: all the ingredients of crispy bread. This meant that she would not be allowed to eat cheese pies, pita bread, or any of the other goodies that made our visits to Greece so special. She could not eat cookies, cakes, or other sweets, ice cream in a cone, pizzas, or pasta made with those ingredients.

If the biopsy showed that Danai's body was badly affected by food containing gluten, she would have to be on a special diet for the rest of her life. I wanted to know what the consequences would be for her body if she did not go on this diet. The doctor explained that she would stop growing. It would be as if her body was not nourished at all. In a person with celiac disease, the interior of the small intestine is sensitive to gluten, which flattens the surface until it cannot retain any amount of food. I had never heard of anything like this before, and once more was in shock.

How could I tell my child that she could not enter a bakery in Greece and get one of her favorite snacks? How could I tell her that she could not have pasta at our favorite Italian restaurant, or ever again eat pita bread, the favorite of all Greeks, when we went to a souvlaki place? The doctor must have heard my broken voice and desperation. He must have felt my immense sorrow. I heard him say that nothing was certain yet—the results of the biopsy would give us a clearer picture. Before our conversation ended, there was one last thing I wanted the doctor to tell me. How valid was the blood test? It was correct sixty percent of the time, he said.

My defense mechanism began to interfere. I wanted
to convince myself that Danai belonged to the forty
percent whose blood tests raised the suspicion of
gluten intolerance but whose biopsies showed that
all was well. Despite all the turmoil, surely there
would be no indication of celiac disease. I wanted to
believe that Danai had nothing to do with this sort of
complication, an extra burden on her already
burdened soul. I could not just accept that we—and
especially Danai—had received another heavy blow.
Many "whys" flooded my stream of thought. Hadn't
we worked hard to manage her diabetes? Hadn't we
met the multiple demands of diabetes with great
bravery and generosity? Wasn't all this hardship
enough? Was the first trial not enough for this child?
Why? The doctor and I agreed that we would wait
until after her birthday party to let her know what
was happening.

The most special day of the year arrived, the day that
every child waits for in great anticipation. Danai did
not have the slightest idea what was happening in
her body. My husband and I were the only ones who
knew that it was the last time she would enjoy a
birthday cake containing gluten, the last birthday
when she would eat her favorite bread and spaghetti
dishes without worrying about anything apart from
matching the carbohydrates she consumed to the
right amount of injected insulin. It was a birthday
when I was trying to hide my sorrow and questions,
and the immense inner emptiness I felt while giving

the children what they expected on such a day. It was an otherwise joyful time and Danai felt proud and happy because she had finally turned twelve, leaving the eleventh year of her life behind, reason enough to feel a bit grown up.

After the echoes of the birthday party had passed, I began to wonder who should talk to her about the new developments—and when and how that should happen. Although I thought about it so many times, from my own perspective as a trusted, familiar person, a mother who talks to her child about everything and always wants the best for her, I still postponed the moment of talking to Danai face-to-face. I did not feel psychologically prepared or ready to do it in a way that would give her the necessary confidence to face an extra challenge. I let the time pass, as Danai's scheduled diabetic check-up was approaching. I tried to convince myself that the doctor should talk to her, while I pretended I was hearing about it for the first time.

However, this sort of arrangement did not satisfy me. I did not want her to find herself exposed to another serious trial, without my having prepared her, even a little. Gradually, I began to realize that, once again, I had to grit my teeth and tell her—or at least hint—that her latest blood test had showed she needed further medical examinations in the hospital. At the same time, I did not want her to drag this worrying piece of information around for a prolonged period of time. I did not want her to worry at school, at home, or when she was walking down the street. I did not want to prolong her agony any more than was absolutely necessary. For all of these reasons, I waited until just a few hours before our meeting with the doctor to tell Danai that our familiar ritual would be different this time because the doctor would talk to us about a special medical examination that had to be carried out.

The diabetologist's outpatient appointments were always on Mondays. Another Monday trial. Another manic Monday? Did we always have to learn about new challenges on Monday? On the other hand, what difference did it make? I will never forget any of the days on which we heard a diagnosis or any serious announcement, no matter how long ago or when they happened. When we arrived at the hospital, the nurses carried out the initial stages of Danai's diabetes checkup. Then her doctor arrived, positioning himself, as always, in his desk chair, while we—Danai, my husband and I—waited on the other side of the desk. Danai and I exchanged smiling glances, as we always did, saying to one another in Greek that the doctor was still wearing the same shoes. We could see them under his desk: they were brown, with some kind of woven pattern on top, and definitely made of leather. I always thought those shoes must be very comfortable to wear—the right footwear for the demands of his job, having to walk up and down the hospital corridors all day long.

This man, the diabetologist, was a professional. Only he knew how many times in the course of his career he had been in this position—sitting opposite families like ours, waiting to make an announcement. Only he knew how many times he had had to tell a diabetic child that she had to go back into the hospital for another three days to be tested for celiac disease, and what it all meant. I cannot otherwise explain the indifference with which he delivered his message. Having to spend three days in the hospital was the first upsetting news. Danai could not process all the new information fast enough to appreciate what it would mean for her in the long run. Three days in the hospital was absolutely necessary to go through the whole process, including the special diabetes care she would need. The doctor gave us a date to present ourselves, and then the meeting was over.

Once more, I adopted the role of psychological consoler. I started thinking up arguments for why the whole experience would be beneficial for Danai. I told her that it was very important to secure her physical integrity and that this had to be our priority. I did not need to mention her initial reactions of denial, sadness, and anger. I expected these and considered them natural. I thought it was good that Danai at least felt free to express her negative emotions, given all she had to tolerate. We told her teacher which days she would have to miss school and why, and we prepared ourselves for another hospital admission.

Meanwhile, I began to prepare Danai for the probable outcome: that she would not be able to eat certain foods any more. At the same time, I pointed out to her the many different alternatives that were available to help people live with this complication. After talking to the doctor on the phone before her birthday, I had found in a bookshop a surprisingly large selection of books on gluten-free cooking. I had also seen on supermarket shelves a considerable range of gluten-free products. These became my weapons in this new battle, reassuring me that we would be back on our feet again fast. The plethora of gluten-free products also made me think there must be many people living with the same problem, whether or not they were type one diabetics. Many times in the past, the thought that I was not alone on this planet facing a problem had helped me, reducing my pain and giving me the strength to go on. It helped me when we were in the airport on our first flight to Greece, when I saw how the luggage controllers handled the fact that one of us was diabetic. The same thought also helped when I was breastfeeding my children all through the night and felt—although I did it with love—exhausted. When I was studying for hours on end in the middle of the night during my time at university, knowing that I was not the only person in this particularly demanding situation was a relief. Such thoughts always make me

feel that I am in the imaginary company of thousands
of fellow-strugglers—and company (good company)
makes me happy.

23. IN THE HOSPITAL ONCE AGAIN

Danai's room in the diabetes ward was reserved days in advance, even before she was admitted to the hospital. She had to undergo her examination in this department for obvious reasons. Danai shared her room with a younger girl, who had been admitted with a liver problem. I was surprised to see how naturally and easily she explained to her roommate and her roommate's parents why she was in the hospital. Perhaps being among children who were facing other serious problems, some even more serious than diabetes and celiac disease, helped her adopt this attitude. Danai was not the only child scheduled for a biopsy. The little girl in her room was there for the same examination and that helped. It also helped that I had told Danai about having a similar experience myself in the past; on that occasion, I had not felt any pain. She saw me being confident—convinced that such medical examinations were necessary for her health. She heard my reassurances that all would go well and waited patiently for her turn to come.

The day after her hospital admission was a crucial one. The biopsy would be carried out under general anesthesia. Avoiding any diabetes-related complications was one of the experts' responsibilities. From early in the morning that day, we waited for it to be Danai's turn. She would not be brought to an ordinary operating room, but to a room on the ground floor of the hospital, which was specially equipped for such procedures. The little girl with the liver problem was taken in before Danai. In the examination room, we were told, there would be an anesthetist, a pediatrician, a diabetologist, a gastroenterologist, nurses, and many apparatuses. I saw all this when a nurse came and announced that it was time to go downstairs, at the same time releasing the brakes on Danai's bed, so that she could push it out of the room.

Danai was composed and surprisingly calm, looking at me for reassurance, and I signaled back the messages she needed to receive. I told her there was no reason for her to worry, that doctors perform such examinations on children many times a day and it would soon be over. Meanwhile, her bed was approaching the elevator. Once more, I tried to raise my daughter's spirits, without letting her know how upset I was. I was watching her lie in bed with tubes in her hands and arms, with the permanent burden of diabetes. I was watching her make heroic efforts to be brave one more time, and I did not want her to know how hard the whole situation was for me.

The nurse who happened to be working that shift and had the job of escorting us to the biopsy room ruined our efforts to cope with the situation. While the elevator was going down, I stood behind Danai's bed so that she would not see the tears on my face. I allowed myself to cry and let my feelings go until we reached the ground floor. I knew I would have enough time, walking behind Danai's bed as we came out of the elevator and headed toward our destination, to dry my tears, straighten up, and begin encouraging her again. However, while the elevator was moving, out of the blue the nurse decided to inform the patient that now they would have to find a way to console her mother. This inconsiderate and inappropriate comment not only surprised me, it also made Danai turn around to see my reaction. The result of all this was that she began to worry about her own condition.

However, we both had to get over this incident really fast; another one followed soon after, which was even tougher to face. We had reached the room where the biopsy would take place and the anesthetist, after introducing himself, told me I could stay with my daughter until the narcotic began to affect her. Danai felt uncomfortable having so many doctors around her. Their presence made her feel that her condition was serious. To me it was reassuring that so many experts were there with her, and I told her so. She held my hand and I felt how worried she was, despite not wanting others to know. The anesthetist introduced himself to his patient and explained what he was about to do. He reassured me that her blood sugar levels would be under control throughout the whole process to avoid hypoglycemia. I was sure that all of these people would perform their tasks competently, but I still felt worried. After a while, when Danai was under the influence of the narcotic, someone led me out of the room and told me they would contact me and my husband, who had just arrived, as soon as they were finished. Now that my child was asleep, my face was flooded with tears.

If I remember correctly, the door of the operation room opened an hour later, when the anesthetist came out to tell us that everything had gone well and the whole process had been a success. When we went in to talk to the gastroenterologist about the outcome, we found Danai sleeping and the doctors putting away their equipment. The gastroenterologist approached us holding pictures, which confirmed that the small intestine had been affected by celiac disease through the consumption of gluten. From now on, Danai would have to go on a strict diet to eliminate that ingredient.

However, that was not the whole diagnosis. A sample of her small intestine would be sent away for a biopsy. I began to hope that perhaps the laboratory results would allow her to go on eating her favorite foods. Once again, I went through the process of denial, as I had when she was first diagnosed with diabetes. I did not want to believe that our reality was being turned upside down again. How much more would this brave girl have to endure? I hoped deeply that something could be done to give this new challenge a more agreeable aspect. I did not want to think about how difficult it would be for Danai to accept additional restrictions to her already demanding life with diabetes.

A few days later, we received the biopsy result. As it was positive, we were immediately given an appointment with the hospital nutritionist. We had to show up for an information session on how to live with celiac disease. The brave girl now asked to make one more big compromise quickly acknowledged that, despite all the problems she was facing, she was still leading a good life, especially compared with the millions of people in other parts of the world who daily starve and face all kinds of other hardships. This twelve-year-old girl was asked once more to demonstrate bravery and strength and to accept that from now on she could not eat what other children ate in school, at the neighborhood bakery, or at her favorite restaurants. I am not at all sure that I could have faced this additional difficulty with as much courage and composure as Danai did from the start.

24. NEW CHANGES AND EFFORTS TO ADJUST

Celiac disease was the next challenge we had to face, through flexible thinking and quick adjustments. A few days after Danai's diagnosis, we found ourselves back on the ground floor of the hospital for our meeting with the nutritionist. This time it was a young woman, not the specialist who had talked to us some years before about living with diabetes. The minute we entered her office, she spread out a number of plastic food samples on her desk and started talking about celiac disease.

We did not know that we could not use our old wooden spoons for cooking, because gluten cannot be washed off wood no matter how hard you try. During that meeting, we also learned that we would have to use separate spreads for bread to avoid the danger of contaminating Danai's food with gluten. I was particularly surprised to learn that we had to be careful even with shampoo, as some contain gluten, which can get into the blood through the skin. For the same reason, Danai had to avoid direct contact with any products containing gluten, such as dough or plasteline. The nutritionist told us to be very conscientious when we wiped the table to make sure that Danai's body never came into contact with gluten.

When the meeting ended, I felt the additional burden of this new responsibility. I wondered how many more times we would need to react, like the butterflies of Manchester, in order to survive. No matter how confident I tried to be in coping with this additional restriction to Danai's life, I could not avoid thinking that, once again, I could not reverse a situation that was causing her discomfort. Now we not only had to weigh her food, but also to cook it very precisely, paying extra attention to everything we did. However, the new diagnosis did not upset me as much as the diabetes diagnosis had. My encounter with diabetes had trained me to adjust quickly and without fatalism to remarkable life changes.

None of us in the family intended to give in to this new turn of events. We all wanted to discover alternative solutions and ways to adjust quickly to this challenge. I read on the Internet that, while one in a thousand people living in the West used to suffer from celiac disease, the current figure is one in a hundred-and-forty. This was another piece of information that helped me pick up the pieces and move on. It helped to know that Danai was not the only person in the world with this peculiar condition.

Before we even met the nutritionist at the hospital, I had already bought gluten-free cookies, flour, and noodles. My purpose was to demonstrate to Danai that there was a solution to the new problem. I already knew that gluten-free products should be kept separate from products that contain gluten. I had read on the Internet and in books that from now on we would have to strictly separate the two. Just as I had to find space to store Danai's diabetic equipment four years earlier, I now had to find space to store the gluten-free flours, noodles, and whatever else we had bought her to eat. This time I emptied a kitchen drawer and, after cleaning it thoroughly, used it to store food that was now exclusively Danai's.

In the same spirit, I bought a rolling pin and started making bread, pizza dough, noodles, and sweets that were gluten-free, something that filled her with joy. Additionally, we bought new wooden spoons for cooking, as we had been instructed to do. We take these with us whenever we stay with friends for a longer period of time. We cook noodles in two different pots and Danai uses her own spread on gluten-free bread. We stopped going to the Italian restaurant in the neighborhood, but continued to go to the Indian restaurant, where most of the food was naturally gluten-free. We searched and found different sources of gluten-free products. Very quickly, we discovered that our favorite pizzeria also offered gluten-free pizza; as I am filling up these pages with our adventures, I should say that we have been positively surprised a number of times. The bistro in our neighborhood is run by an Italian woman and offers gluten-free soups, pizza, and noodles. Two days ago, we read in the local newspaper that a new bakery had opened ten miles from home, exclusively making gluten-free bread and other goodies. In addition, a frozen food home delivery service provides us with ice cream cones, pizza, and bread—all gluten-free.

I was particularly happy to discover on the Internet a pastry shop in Athens that not only made gluten-free cheese pies, a favorite among most Greeks, but also produced a variety of gluten-free sweets. Without delay, I got in touch with the owner, to make sure it was true. Not only do many wonderful people provide celiacs with a wide range of tasty products, those products are in high demand all over the country, proving that the statistics on the growing number of people needing gluten-free nutrition are correct. I immediately told Danai the happy news; the Greek pastry shop will certainly be one of the first places we visit on our next trip to Athens. I felt that my child's patience was being rewarded in one way or another. I kept reminding Danai that the most important thing was to take good care of her body, because life is much more than just what we eat. I also reminded her that the purpose of being alive was not to consume food—we consume food in order to stay alive, something she had already learned from her previous experiences.

25. AN AGGRAVATION FOR THE FAMILY: THE REACTIONS OF OTHER PEOPLE

At this point I would like to appeal to people who have not been affected by the demands, challenges, difficulties, and dangers of diabetes—those who have not crossed its threshold of permanent hardships, but who are, for some reason, reading this book.

Every family with a child who bears the burden of a type one diabetes diagnosis faces psychological fluctuations and practical adversities on a daily basis. For this reason, it would be helpful if others could become aware that diabetes-related comments of any sort made on behalf of third parties can seriously upset and even harm the members of the diabetic family.

Comments can cause harm even if they are not intended to. I therefore recommend approaching diabetic families with special care, as well as tolerance, understanding, open-mindedness, patience, and discretion. It is equally important not to confront the diabetic child and his or her family with poisonous and soul-destroying expressions of pity, the negative effects of which I have already discussed. People who sincerely wish to offer support and help should make an honest decision about how to contribute in a positive way to the life of the diabetic family.

I feel a need to bring this up because of incidents that have occurred from the time of Danai's diabetes diagnosis until the present day—experiences that have hurt and greatly disappointed me. During these five years, while we were struggling to come to terms with our new reality, I noticed changes in the behavior of people in our social circle. Their reactions made me feel intensely that my family and I were becoming marginalized. I observed that the harder we worked to reconcile ourselves to the new challenges, the less tolerant people around us became in accepting the new terms and conditions of our life. The non-diabetic world seemed unable or unwilling to understand that the new turn our lives had taken was absolutely essential and mandatory. I could see that most of the people we had shared our lives with up to then did not want to understand or cooperate with the necessarily strict life schedule we had to follow, with set lunch and dinner times and injections of insulin. As a result, we saw less and less of our so-called friends. Their phone calls, which I had the impression were mostly acts of curiosity, also decreased over time. For Danai, sleeping over at friends' homes was difficult and many times impossible. One particularly unfortunate circumstance made her feel rejected: her best friend did not invite Danai to her birthday party because, "you are diabetic." It was the first proof that what I was observing was not just a figment of my imagination.

Another incident that exemplified our experiences as a diabetic family was the reaction of a woman who invited us to dinner. What followed this invitation not only stifled Danai, but also Ioli and me. This woman had shown some understanding of our special needs as a diabetic family, but her sympathy decreased considerably as the evening progressed. The final straw was her obvious despair at the prospect of having to wait for a few minutes (so that Danai's insulin could take effect) before satisfying her own instinct for self-preservation by consuming all the goodies she'd prepared for dinner. This was one of the experiences that changed my attitude about social gatherings. I promised myself that we would stop experimenting. It would be better to stay at home for lunch and dinner, or at least to socialize only with people who did not make our already difficult lives even more difficult.

I did not see why we should spend time with people who could not understand what it meant to live with type one diabetes. There was no reason, I thought, to victimize and impose our strict rules on so many innocent people. Or was this a good opportunity to separate our real friends from mere acquaintances? I took the opportunity and did exactly that. So there was a benefit, after all. Diabetes was useful for more than just mental invigoration. In relief, I concluded that diabetes could help to clear away meaningless and damaging human contacts. It helped us separate the wheat from the chaff. Not bad at all.

The hurtful comments did not stop when Danai received her second diagnosis of celiac disease. The sad thing in all of this was that the harder we worked—especially Danai—to adjust to one more challenge and change, the more people's reactions weighed us down. The "Ohh, another problem?" sort of reaction, egocentricity at its best, which made me feel as if someone was hammering my head, re-emerged, causing havoc. At that point, I could not and was not willing to tolerate a chorus of new voices expressing "sorrow." I did not want and could not stand watching people become overexcited, as if their own lives were under threat because Danai´s body was gluten-sensitive and needed insulin.

I could not and did not want to deal with the superficial interest expressed by people who constantly gave priority to their own needs and did not give a damn how we really felt. I did not want more promises of contact or invitations to lunch or dinner that never materialized. Who would bother with dinner invitations and human contact when most people are drawn into the swirl of their own egoism? The process of marginalization was alive and kicking.

In extreme cases, people's comments far exceeded the limits of my tolerance. As an example, I will mention our last visit to the dentist: an unpleasant moment caused by the reaction of a self-centered, inconsiderate being.

Our dentist, in addition to being very good at his job, has a natural kindness and a positive attitude toward life. There is nothing fake about him. On the contrary, he listens to our problems with compassion and sincerity. He does whatever he can do to boost my morale. For this reason, I cannot explain how such a gentle and cultivated person can employ such a heartless assistant to treat his patients' teeth.

The children came into contact with this woman during a routine checkup: first Danai, who decided to go into the treatment room on her own, and then Ioli, who went in with me. From my point of view, this dental assistant already had a criminal record after making an unacceptable and incredibly inhuman comment about Danai's diabetes during our previous visit. My daughter had come out of the dental assistant's office obviously shocked to tell me what had happened. I initially wanted to talk to her employer, our dentist, but I did not want to trouble or upset him. I decided to ignore the incident and not to mention it to him or reprimand his assistant.

My generosity ended when it was Ioli's turn in the chair. I had asked whether the substances she was using to protect the children's teeth contained gluten. With a look of satisfaction, the dental assistant threw back the most inappropriate and tasteless question:

"Die hat ja alles, oder? (she has everything, doesn't she?)."

It wasn't just her provocative comment, but the pleasure she obviously took in uttering it. Her face glowed; her smile confirmed how much she enjoyed the suffering of others. Despite this fatal combination of reactions, she dared to look me in the eye without a trace of shame.

I wonder whether there is any mother in this world who could ignore such a bitter comment. Some minutes earlier, the dental assistant had been describing her own (obesity-related) health problems, explaining that she could not swim because of her physique and only walked in the sea when she was on vacation. Instead of putting me in my place, her comment made me furious. I think she forgot that I was equipped with the world's most effective shield: motherhood.

My firm reaction was the perfect antidote. The dental assistant's attitude changed instantly. She tried to convince me with a fake, hypocritical smile that her intentions were good, that I did not need to talk to her employer, and that she understood and would be more careful when we next met on a purely professional basis. The irony was that Danai, who was off to her weekly badminton lesson after her appointment, was actually healthier than this immobile, self-centered creature.

This incident was one of those moments when I was forced to defend myself to stop outsiders interfering with my child's private life. It was a moment when I refused to apologize for our way of life. Although I was careful to protect my daughter before our next visit, I had been forced to invest valuable energy in dealing with something unpleasant— energy that should have been used to do something revitalizing and creative. As we came out of the dentist's office,

Danai asked me to mention this incident in my book, to help others empathize with the millions of people with special needs who live around them.

After the second diagnosis, I had to spend valuable energy resisting many people's exaggerated reactions and reassuring them that our lives were not over, and particularly Danai's, just because her eating habits had changed. In addition to those rare friends who expressed genuine interest and love, those who faced similar challenges for themselves or their families were our best support: able to understand and accept that our way of living was different but nevertheless viable.

26. FROM INJECTIONS TO THE PUMP: A HIGHLY DESIRABLE CHANGE

No matter how hard one works to adjust to cantankerous diabetes and escape its limitations, the daily routine of the diabetic child remains demanding. My experiences during the five years Danai has lived with diabetes make me believe that insulin injections considerably added to the physical pain she felt and the psychological hurdles she encountered. As I have already mentioned, Danai had insulin injections for almost five years. For most of that time, she perceived the moment of the injection as a dreadful routine.

 Danai's physical growth imposed a change on the quantity and frequency of her insulin injections. While initially needing two injections of insulin daily, in time she ended up injecting five or six times a day. As her daily demand for insulin increased, so did her pain, despair, discomfort, and other uncomfortable feelings. Not only Danai, but our whole family became embroiled in this ordeal.

At the same time, natural hormonal variations began to influence the effect of insulin on her body. As a result, Danai's blood sugar levels fluctuated frenetically. For a long time, we lived in a diabetic paradox, taking care of her hypoglycemic state almost every midnight, and then measuring dangerously high levels of sugar in her blood in the morning. These fluctuations not only caused physical discomfort, but also affected Danai psychologically. A troubling side-effect was that Danai began to suffer from sleeping disorders. "Why should I sleep? You are going to wake me up anyway," she told me one night when I found her staring at the ceiling with eyes wide open, waiting for her father or me to come in and prick her fingers. Multiple hypoglycemic incidents caused her to gain weight as she was forced to consume carbohydrates to rebalance her body.

Whenever we met Danai's doctor at the hospital for a scheduled checkup, we described him the situation we were in and expressed our concern about Danai´s well-being. We told him our observations in the hope that he would suggest a way out of this misery and help her body to react more efficiently, reducing her psychological strain. Unfortunately, our ordeal lasted for a long time. The specialist, a university professor, suggested introducing minute and completely ineffective alterations to Danai's insulin intake. For a long period of time, he experimented on her body, changing the type or quantity of insulin she had to inject at night; all of these attempts were completely unproductive. For a long period of time, we entered his office in despair, only to leave it feeling helpless. Although we are not doctors, we could see that the treatments the diabetologist was proposing were not the best on offer.

At the same time, people who had nothing to do with the world of diabetes were giving me information about insulin pumps. My neighbor knew a girl whose diabetes had improved when she started using the pump. The dance school director knew another diabetic girl, an insulin pump user, who had started dancing classes without the constant threat of hypoglycemia. A friend had heard from others about the beneficial effect of the insulin pump on the treatment of diabetes.

It was absolutely urgent that we find a solution to the harmful sugar fluctuations in Danai's blood. Through the use of the pump Danai would stop the painful and repulsive multiple daily injections and get a better life. So we began visiting the doctor, equipped with this supporting information and hinting at our wish to change Danai's treatment. Unfortunately, the diabetologist was not of the same school of thought, although a number of his colleagues were. For a long time, all of our efforts to communicate with him proved futile. For reasons we never understood, he tried to discourage us from seeking this alternative solution. He asked us to explain how Danai could go swimming if she had a pump, almost seeming to reverse the doctor-patient relationship. We had to come up with arguments to convince him to approve the use of a pump. His consent was essential; without it, our health insurance would not finance the pump.

Every time we visited the doctor, we had to tell him that his suggestions for regulating Danai's diabetes weren't working. As we hoped he would agree to provide her with an insulin pump, we ended up feeling that he did not give a damn about her health. Again and again, he just signed, in his familiar, sluggish way, a pile of new prescriptions for Danai. They were prescriptions for more injections and for hundreds of new syringes to pierce her body with their delicate little needles, supplying it with either the same or a slightly altered quantity of insulin.

Many times, our meetings left my husband and me with an unpleasant aftertaste. The three of us observed the etiquette of acceptable behavior, making little jokes here and there, being polite to each other, and engaging in small talk. However, I could not help feeling that this doctor wasn't doing everything he could to meet Danai's needs. I suspected that if she had been his own daughter, he would have tried other ways of treating diabetes than the ones he was suggesting to us. As time progressed, I increasingly felt that he was not making a real effort to help. Instead, I had the impression that he was focused on his career at the hospital, which put money in the bank and paid for him and his family to have a very comfortable life. For one thing, it did not seem to bother Danai's doctor that he wasn't succeeding in regulating her diabetes. I couldn't help thinking that he just wasn't concerned about the long-term impact of his ineffective treatments on my child's body.

Over a long period of time, whenever we failed to obtain the doctor's approval for a pump, or left his office without achieving a significant change, I felt like an accomplice to a crime. So we stopped being patient and obedient to the doctor's wishes and changed our tactics. During our scheduled hospital visits, my husband and I told him what we thought

Danai should have. We put pressure on him to find some new way of regulating her diabetes. We knew that she could have the opportunity to experience life with a pump for one weekend (without using it to receive insulin), and this is what we asked for. All we needed to do was organize a meeting with Mrs. In-a-Hurry, the advisor for diabetic families. At that point, the diabetologist finally realized that we were desperately looking for help. He gave his consent for a trial with the pump.

This is how Danai ended up very quickly receiving information on all the different types of insulin pumps available on the market. Although the device was new to her, she was willing to try to live with a pump attached to her body for one weekend. From that moment on, the distant prospect I had asked her to believe in during the days following her diagnosis—that she would not always need to inject insulin—became a potential reality. The possibility that she could regulate her diabetes by using a pump added a note of optimism to our lives. At times when Danai felt resentful, it was possible to think about an alternative, promising aid that could make her life easier in many ways. We held tight to the hope that she could use a pump; from that weekend of testing onwards, we began to smile.

I had the feeling that now I could hope for a future with less turmoil. Meanwhile, the dangerous fluctuations in Danai's blood sugar levels were still giving her body and psyche a hard time. We had to act fast. On our next meeting with her doctor, we told him that we wanted her to have a pump and were ready for her to go back into the hospital to take part in seminars on life with it.

Twice a year, the hospital offered educational seminars on using a pump to type one diabetic children and their parents. We did not want to miss the next training session, which was scheduled to take place very soon. We wanted Danai to start living with fewer problems, with less fear and discomfort. However, here too we ran into a number of obstacles. Her doctor admitted that her case could be treated with the help of the pump, but he was convinced that our health insurance would not cover this kind of treatment because of Danai's HbA1 value. He did not expect me to mistrust his advice or be able to think for myself. However, I knew that the HbA1 value was an average of many blood sugar fluctuations over a period of two to three months. Because it averaged together many high and low blood sugar values, it was unimportant in Danai's case. In other words, an average is useless when the main problem is deregulated diabetes. I questioned the doctor's argument and began to trust him even less than before.

The final blow came when he told us that, if we would agree to take part in some research his own and other universities were conducting on using the insulin pump to improve the lives of diabetic people, he could guarantee that Danai would get a pump without our health insurance interfering. He could not, however, guarantee that Danai would participate in the first group to be investigated. In other words, she might have to wait for six months or even longer to get a pump.

The doctor's attempt to sacrifice our needs as a diabetic family to satisfy his own was a fatal mistake on his part. I felt that we were slowly becoming part of a dirty game. If we did not resist, we would end up being his guinea pigs. I did not want my child's health to become a pawn in the hands of indifferent researchers. We deserved better and we deserved to be taken seriously. We were facing a serious situation. I had heard so much about the pump's benefits for diabetics and I wanted my daughter to have them. The insulin pump is not a fashion accessory. It is not "in" or "out." It is a matter of health—my daughter's physical health. After being under so much pressure, we immediately contacted our health insurance and explained why we were seeking their approval for an alternative way to treat Danai's condition. We also made clear that we needed their authorization as soon as possible.

Fortunately, our health insurance reacted promptly on receiving documentation of Danai's blood sugar measurements. The hormonal fluctuations of puberty are an extra burden in the effort to regulate diabetes, as they interfere with the effect of insulin. Danai's age was one of the health insurance company's decisive reasons for approving the financing so quickly. All of the necessary steps to provide the pump were taken fast, the right reaction to an emergency.

After so many years, things had started to work for us at last. I was happy for Danai and grateful to everyone at our health insurance company for taking her case seriously, even without having known her personally for many years, as her doctor had. A few days later, Danai's name appeared on the list of candidates receiving an insulin pump from the diabetes ward of the children's hospital. This is how the three of us (Danai and her parents) participated in educational seminars offered by the hospital to learn how to operate the pump.

Although my husband and I were happy that the big change had finally arrived and was promising to improve her quality of life, Danai was in a huff. Her admission to the hospital was scheduled to take place during the summer vacation, so that it would not interfere with school. Danai could not see why she should spend part of her precious break in the hospital. I sympathized with her. I don't know any child who would want to exchange sun and vacation relaxation for several days in the hospital, especially when that child has been through this experience a number of times already. However, it was something that had to be done. Danai had to sacrifice part of her summer vacation on the altar of health.

But that was not the only thing that upset her. She was uncomfortable with the idea that she would always have something attached to her body that would be visible to others. She worried about sleeping, dancing, doing sports, and living life with this plastic piece of equipment attached to her hip. At that point, I asked Danai to name something I carried on my own body—something essential that I was not born with. After looking hard at me for some time, she concluded that it had to be my clothes. Good thinking. Nobody goes around without clothes, although they are pieces of cotton, wool, or man-made material added to our bodies. No one is born with shoes on their feet, although most of us wear shoes, at least outdoors.

But this wasn't what I wanted her to notice. I gave her another chance. "Your watch," she said after observing me for quite some time. Yes, I could not exist without my watch. I am so addicted to it that I wear it every day, even though it can be too heavy for me sometimes. But it wasn't my watch I wanted Danai to notice.

"Danai," I told her, "you are so used to seeing me wear glasses that you didn't even think of mentioning them. My glasses are an awkward appendage that I nevertheless have to carry on my body, and they are visible to everyone around me."

I need and wear glasses, although I don't find them pleasant, especially on rainy or winter days or when I have to take food out of the oven. Although it is taken for granted and socially accepted that some people wear glasses, I have never met anyone who was overjoyed to have vision aids sitting on his or her nose. As with all things in life, when you give something, you get something in return. This is what I wanted Danai to realize. By allowing the pump to operate on her body, she would receive its benefits.

Danai had to get used wearing the pump, just as an untamed horse has to get used to his saddle. She had to be able to wear it without feeling inhibited or insecure and without worrying about how it looked or what other people might think. During that transitory period of her life, it was essential for Danai to give herself time to adjust to this challenge, paving the way for a new life with diabetes. She had to understand that using the pump was the best thing she could do for her physical and psychological health—and not worry about bothering other people. If people were disturbed at the sight of her pump, then that would be another good opportunity to separate the wheat from the chaff. Sometimes I sing her part of an old Greek song, which goes: "we will stick with the ones who like us, we cannot do much for the ones who do not …," and we both laugh.

27. ANOTHER HOSPITAL ADMISSION, THIS TIME BY OUR OWN CHOICE

During our next stay in the hospital, we spent ten days attending seminars on the use of the pump, helping Danai's body adapt to this alternative way of treating her diabetes. Our group consisted of children and teenagers between five and eighteen years of age, as well as their parents, all there for the same reason. A few days after we received the green light from our health insurance company, the familiar images and smells of the hospital were around us once more. Figures dressed in white came in and out of rooms. From various parts of the ward came shrieking machine sounds and the whole hospital environment reminded me of everything we had experienced so many times before.

Wasn't the hospital our second home by now? Its beds, our beds? Its kitchen, our kitchen? Why not? Sometimes I told the children that we should not be afraid of the hospital, but should think of it as a place where necessary help is offered. This time, we had asked for the help we were going to receive. We did not have to be there, but we wished to. We wanted Danai to acquire a wider spectrum of freedoms, as was appropriate for a thirteen-year-old girl whom we knew we could absolutely trust. She had to feel free to challenge herself, take the initiative, participate in school excursions, do sports, go to the movies without having to inject insulin in the dark and live life to the full, with less pain and fear.

Those ten days spent in the hospital were a pleasant surprise. It was good to experience it as a place that would help us achieve a better future. It was good to live in there in tranquility, with clear minds and an understanding that we could profit from the benefits this place had to offer. Everything was nicely organized and the staff was friendly. Some days before our admission, we met with a diabetologist who advised families and with a representative of the company providing the pump. During that meeting, we were delighted to find that the atmosphere of the diabetes ward had significantly improved. Mrs. In-a-Hurry, the diabetic families' advisor, had left the hospital. Her replacement was a gentle, patient, compassionate and smiling woman, who was eager to help and always did her best to solve problems that arose.

The three diabetologists leading the seminars were alert and eager to answer all our questions. Danai's doctor was not among them and could not be, since he consistently opposed the use of the pump to treat diabetes. Initially, the family advisor wanted to know what kind of worries, thoughts, and expectations each member of the group had. The doctors wanted to know how long each family had been living with diabetes and how we expected the pump to change our lives.

We began to receive information on life with a pump and about the various qualities and functions of different sorts of insulin. We were told about the thresholds of hyperglycemia and hypoglycemia, and how they would change in these new circumstances, moving toward a healthier framework. Danai's body had to adjust to the new conditions and learn to tolerate lower levels of sugar in her blood without extra care. Everything we heard sounded good. Even before we started living with the pump, or rather, before Danai started living with it, we were overcome with euphoria. The weight Danai had shouldered all these years was finally growing lighter.

The children and young people in our group, or in some cases, their parents, had selected different sorts of pumps for different reasons; these were adjusted to their bodies during the second day of our stay in the hospital. The doctors and advisor supervised each case separately. The fact that the experts were interested in every child, attended to each patient's needs and varying reactions with special care, and were willing to help every diabetic person in the group if the first contact with the pump caused any problems gave me a very positive feeling. I noticed the way the medical staff respected these children's special needs. They seemed fully aware of the distress the new situation was causing both diabetics and their parents.

In the seminar room, I felt that all of us parents had something in common: shared problems, worries, pain, fears, and hopes. As the children and young people were different ages, they reacted differently when the moment came to adjust the pumps on their bodies. While a five-year-old boy panicked and resisted the needle that pierced his belly to allow the tube to be adjusted, an eighteen-year-old did this himself, quite confidently, giving me the impression that he would manage the mechanism of his pump as efficiently as he managed his mobile phone. While the parents of the five-year-old boy were exclusively responsible for operating their son's pump, the eighteen-year-old was unescorted, adjusting his pump calmly and perhaps even with a sense of accomplishment. I felt sure that it had been his decision to seek a better future by adopting an alternative way of treating his diabetes.

Danai, at thirteen years old, benefited from being part of this group. She watched all of the participants' varying reactions. It seemed to me that this team was helping her, perhaps unconsciously, to reorient herself. She could appreciate where she was standing, where she was heading, and how she wanted to proceed with diabetes. It was a chance for her to think about how receptive and open she was willing to be towards this new way of living with her condition. It was equally important for Danai to attend seminars with kids who were facing the same problems, demands, and worries, and feeling the same pain. She shared a classroom with other diabetic children and teenagers who, like herself, were hoping to improve their lives through the use of an insulin pump. I believe that this peer group helped her accept the fact that she would be carrying the pump on her body faster than I had expected, after all the discussions and resistance that had preceded our hospital stay.

The functioning of this remarkable apparatus was tightly supervised in the hospital, once it was adjusted to Danai's body. Her blood sugar levels were monitored regularly, and the doctors made small alterations to the quantity of insulin she received through the pump. However, it was important to bear in mind that hospital living conditions did not reproduce normal life outside. In the hospital, there is almost no physical activity and children experience no school stress—and in particular, no exam stress.

A day or two after Danai began living with the pump, I asked her to estimate how many injections she had already avoided through this wonderful invention. I saw her face brightening with joy and pleasure after a quick calculation, as she realized that from that point onwards, she would not experience the daily threat of injecting insulin. When we returned home, Danai found in the kitchen cupboard the glass container we used to hold used syringes before we threw them away. With relief, she showed me all of the old syringes squeezed into the glass. She asked me what she should do with them. Throw them away, of course! We had to believe that we had entered another era and found a less arduous way to treat diabetes. We had to believe it was time to celebrate a triumph—the moment we had been waiting for so long.

At this point, some parents reading about the way we chose to treat Danai's diabetes may feel that I am suggesting that our choice was better than the way their own children are being treated, if they are still injecting insulin. One should bear in mind that there are a number of factors that influence a doctor's and family's assessment of whether or not a particular child should receive insulin through a pump. These include the age and gender of the child and the family's way of life. An essential condition is that both sides, the doctor and the family, agree that the child would profit from a change in diabetes treatment and be ready for that change.

In the hospital, we spent many hours with the parents and children in our group. We became close to some of them and shared experiences of life with diabetes. It was then that I began to take an idea I had had for a long time—to write this book—very seriously. The trigger was the reaction of one mother in our group. This woman initially seemed to have adopted a very relaxed and accommodating attitude towards her five-year-old son's diabetes. She did not allow the slightest indication of weakness to show in her face. When it was her son's turn to be put on the pump, he protested and resisted. I observed his mother's reactions and assumed that she had fully accepted her child's condition. She seemed to have a reserve of inner strength and composure, which influenced her attitude towards life.

However, I was wrong. A little later, I discovered that the mother of the five-year-old boy had learned to hide her real feelings very well. She had learned to not allow others to see how she really felt about her diabetic son. Her behavior gave me the impression that she had learned, consciously or unconsciously, that it was a mistake to express distress or pain, or to admit how insecure you felt, let tears roll down your face, or dare to show your real self. She must have learned that such behavior could be taken for weakness, dangerously exposing you to others. This woman did not want the people around her to think she was a weak mother, perhaps because she knew how strong she had to appear next to her five-year-old diabetic son.

I realized that the mother of the diabetic boy was suppressing her feelings when we started talking privately in her son's room. During our discussion, she let the pain surface and become visible on her face just for a little while; her eyes filled with tears and her voice was tremulous. When I felt she was letting her guard down, I grasped the opportunity and signaled that it was not sinful to talk about negative emotions. Instead, it was important to allow them to be part of one's reality. My reassurances helped her be more honest with herself and let negative emotions come to the surface. I had no right to judge her but I felt for her. It was the human reaction of someone who needed help and immediate psychological support. I had been living with my child's diagnosis of diabetes for five years and had learned a lot during that time. She had only lived with her son's diagnosis for a year and still had a lot to learn.

I offered her my help and she accepted it. I talked about ways to stop the self-destructive behavior she was engaging in. I wanted her to see that what she and her son were going through was a life lesson, and that she should focus less on the diabetes itself. She was wasting precious time in unbearable pain. I hoped that she would realize that her son was radiating with an amazing energy and strength. Presumably, her sorrow made it hard for her to see his true potential. I urged her not to treat him as someone sick and weak, but to offer him the opportunity to develop fully, in accordance with his talents and intelligence, which were both remarkable. While I tried to help this mother escape her grief, I could see that her son was charming everybody in the diabetes ward with his strong and charismatic personality. So I asked her to turn around and look at him, and to consider whether it was fair to think of him as an invalid.

I felt and saw that my words were not wasted and that something had begun to improve in this mother's inner world. She smiled, appearing to appreciate the new perspective that had begun to take shape in front of her eyes. I interpreted her reaction as a sign that she was willing to change the way she was treating her diabetic son. Just at that moment, in the corridor of the hospital diabetes ward, she seemed to have adopted a brand-new way of thinking that was likely to last.

That impression was confirmed the next morning, when she approached me on her own initiative and asked me to repeat what I had told her the day before, when I was trying to boost her morale, "as it had all been so helpful." I smiled, and let her know that I was thinking of finally writing the book I had been mulling over for a long time. Her enthusiasm about this idea helped to persuade me to sit down and write this book.

28. A NEW START WITH THE INSULIN PUMP

A long time has passed since our voluntary stay in the hospital. Changing the way Danai treats her diabetes has helped her lead a less troublesome life, although we continue to cooperate with her doctor in order to achieve even better results. During her stay in the hospital, Danai decided not to keep seeing the specialist she was initially allocated to. Instead, she chose one of the female diabetologists—partly because she was a woman, but mainly because she reacted to Danai's needs immediately, inspiring trust.

Although the insulin pump is a valuable tool for the diabetic child, it cannot replace the functions of a healthy pancreas by 100%. The pump is not an artificial pancreas, but just the best human invention available to keep blood sugar values at an acceptable level much of the time, in the least painful way possible. Although the pump is not a perfect solution to the riddle of type one diabetes, its benefits are numerous and remarkable. Danai can regulate the amount of insulin flowing into her body during and after physical activities. As a result, she is not hypoglycemic as often as she used to be, an essential ingredient for physical and psychological balance.

An additional beneficial outcome is a reduction in the frequent hyperglycemic incidents she used to have during the night and in the early morning. In a boost to Danai's moral, the bruises have disappeared from the injection sites on her body; these were an almost permanent side effect of insulin injections. She derives great pleasure from having more freedom to decide when and how much she will eat, provided she eats at regular intervals. We have all benefited from this new treatment because it has allowed us to stop panicking about making sure that Danai eats at strictly determined time intervals, something that created a great deal of stress during the first five years.

Danai very quickly accepted the presence of the insulin pump, which usually hangs over her trousers.

She learned to operate it equally fast. Now, managing the pump is her own almost exclusive responsibility, providing her with increased autonomy. Since we came back from the hospital, I have only rarely had to sit beside her and console her or cheer her up. Instead, we hug each other and talk about how much better things are now; I see her face filled with satisfaction, as she agrees with my positive assessment. I tell Danai how grateful I am to the people who invented this amazing device, the insulin pump—people I will probably never meet. What makes me particularly happy is the fact that she does not make any effort to hide her pump from public view. I deduce from this that she accepts and respects herself the way she is. Such an attitude is precious for her and her future development.

Danai is now in high school. After the summer break, we told her teachers about the change in the way she would be treating her diabetes, sending each of them a letter with a detailed description of this change and what it meant. Her class counselor expressed genuine interest and contacted us to learn in more detail about the treatment of diabetes and Danai's special needs. This teacher says that she admires Danai for her courage and ability to manage the demands of diabetes. She expresses sincere interest in her general condition, and reacts promptly whenever Danai feels unwell. At such times, this teacher always contacts us, making us feel that our child is in good hands.

29. FIVE YEARS LATER

I am not always strong: my own refuge

From the day Danai was diagnosed with type one diabetes to the present, five years have passed. During this period, we have experienced a lot, both as individuals and as a family, and we have also learned a lot from those experiences. The diagnosis threw us into a rough sea of feelings and events. Our love for our child and the desire to help her were the main elements that kept us going. Neither type one diabetes nor celiac disease, with which Danai was diagnosed four years later, will ever leave me indifferent, no matter how many years pass by and no matter how much I try to accept that pain is an ingredient of life. If I want to be honest, I have to admit that diabetes has left a scar. However, the longer I live with it, the less I feel its intensity. The frequency with which I experience negative feelings has also decreased considerably with the passing of time. Today, I consider diabetes to be a part of my child. I no longer cry about it, or walk down the street lost in sorrow and despair.

If someone asked me whether I would choose a life without my daughter's diabetes, given its contribution to my spiritual evolution, I would say yes. Of course, I would want Danai to lead a life without this burden. However, since we are part of this special world we did not choose, and despite its difficulties, we must not miss this opportunity to acknowledge that demanding life situations offer precious lessons.

During five years of living with diabetes, I have managed to change the soul-destroying question, "why did all of this happen to me?" into the more creative and beneficial question, "what can I learn from this?" Every new challenge we face becomes an opportunity to search for and discover something that should not be ignored, a lesson to be learned that will make us stronger. I have learned to think of difficulties as sources of personal wisdom that only the affected individual can discover. I take advantage of life's trials, listening carefully to what they tell me and discovering which spiritual lessons they can teach.

I believe that the challenges Danai faces are an opportunity for her to learn to be tolerant, patient, and hopeful—no matter what she decides to do in life. Danai and I are on this path together. One night, I was giving her an injection before she fell asleep, as I had done thousands of times before. A wave of despair, of psychological exhaustion and pain, seemed to rise from my child's body, hitting each and every one of my own cells. I did not let this sensation discourage me, but chose to see the positive aspects of what we were both experiencing. I searched for a way to take advantage of this pain.

"Danai, you have a lot of power and diabetes has come to make you realize that," I said, in response to the distress I was experiencing. I meant what I was telling her; that was how I felt. Danai did not react to my comment. She neither accepted nor rejected it. Instead, she listened carefully, giving me the impression that somewhere deep inside, she knew that this was a serious and acceptable justification for her body's decision to develop diabetes.

Every time I manage to look Danai's condition straight in the eye, with clarity and without fear, I feel some compensation: my own power increases. The strength I derive from adopting this attitude seems inexhaustible. It is my gift, my reward for dealing courageously with all the ups and downs of our lives. Many times, I have felt that my reserves of psychological strength were endless, unexpectedly immense, as if stored in a barrel without a bottom. They are generously provided each time I manage to be optimistic and make another effort to survive. This strength is the feeling I get each time I overcome another dead end by believing that I can make it through. It is like being magically offered another helping of courage from the bottomless barrel. It is my inner voice telling me that I can manage and will once more find a way to loosen the Gordian knot. It is the voice that tells me I am here to learn and teach my children.

Through the work diabetes forced me to do, I have learned to face difficulties and complications as an integral part of life, while looking for ways to surmount them as quickly as possible. I have learned not to let myself give in to the whirl of negative thoughts. At such moments, I concentrate on possible life scenarios, aiming for the feasible, rather than struggling to achieve the unfeasible. I devote more time to tasting small delights that supply me with new energy. Five years after diabetes brought panic and sorrow, I make plans for the future and organize enjoyable and relaxing activities for the whole family.

As time goes by, I have learned to accept my child's condition, and to live with it; I have integrated it into our daily lives. I do not allow myself to feel sad about the world that collapsed and disappeared. I accept the new and different, which is now our reality. I want to feel complete with what I have. I have a diabetic child with whom I can play hangman, even if we occasionally need to interrupt our game to measure the sugar in her blood. I can play this game and others without thinking about the last time we played before Danai's diagnosis. To survive, I have learned to find alternative ways to achieve our goals, accepting that if we cannot live one way, we will live another way. The important thing is to go on living.

I have learned that diabetes does not have to impede a fully creative, inventive, and humorous life that benefits all involved, and particularly the diabetic child. Many times, I have found that being in a humorous mood helps me find solutions to problems faster, especially when those problems arise from the difficulties and complications of diabetes. Humor makes my life easier. It puts me in the right mood to face challenges in a more effective way. It also helps me lift some of the heavy weight from Danai's shoulders. One morning, as I was driving the children to school, the words of a song on the radio reminded us that, "what does not kill you makes you stronger." I increased the volume so that the refrain could be heard in the back seat as well as the front. I felt grateful to the artists whose message that morning was reinforcing what I was trying to teach my children in my own way.

Considering the seriousness of the problems we face, we are not doing badly at all. However, it took me a considerable amount of time to reach this stage and be able to face problems as I do today. I walked a long path full of lessons, insights, observations, and obstacles, and had long periods of isolation before accepting the new reality. During the first stages of our life with diabetes, when our basic goal was just to survive, I would have resented anyone who tried to talk to me about the benefits of humor. If someone had tried to tell me that life with diabetes was a valuable opportunity to learn to give, be compassionate, and express unconditional love, that message would have seemed inappropriate. Initially, the diabetic child and family are drowning in so many "whys, hows, and whens." They feel intense sorrow, denial, anger, despair, fear, and insecurity. The first moments with diabetes, which must vary in duration and intensity from individual to individual, are moments of rearrangement and reorientation, as people make the effort to accept a new reality. These moments are important, even essential, to the stages that follow. It would be brutal and utopian for an experienced diabetes veteran to demand that a newcomer instantly appreciate everything that others have come to understand only through the passage of time. Messages of support such as: I know what you're going through, I've been through that myself describe an accomplishment that is not negligible, and which can be helpful to diabetic families, even at the beginning of their adventure.

Despite the intensive work I have done on myself over the years, I am not perfect. I am not always strong. Although I don't compare the present to the past as often as I did during our first year with diabetes, I do continue to fall into that trap and probably always will. Fortunately, the intense distress caused by these comparisons has considerably decreased; it does not affect me nearly as much as it did during the first year. I have accepted that comparisons are unavoidable, but I no longer allow them to break me into pieces.

I am not a perfect mother. I am certainly not always a good role model as a mother. I acknowledge my weakness—I can't always face challenges with exemplary determination and sobriety, despite my good intentions. However, I have learned to accept without feeling defeated my human weakness, imperfection, and inability to change every difficult situation that upsets Danai; these are a part of my existence.

There are hundreds of pictures in our family albums taken before the diabetes era, and I accept that these will never leave me indifferent. Although they will never upset me as much as they did immediately after Danai's diagnosis, holding these precious colorful pieces of paper in my hands will always take me back to a past carefree existence, at the seaside, in the mud, in taverns. Through them, the children's voices, laughter, and joy during family gatherings or visits to the zoo will sound louder in my ears; their colors will seem more vivid than they did during the diabetes era. I know I will study my children's beautiful smiles, movements, and trampoline jumps, as well as Danai's first steps and first day at school— all this without being hypoglycemic or having to inject insulin. No matter how often I hold these pictures, or how many years later, they will always remind me that at this or that specific moment, immortalized through the press of a button, Danai was not diabetic. I have decided to give myself the freedom to take such sentimental journeys.

During our five years of symbiosis with type one diabetes, the way I form associations has also changed. This is something I put up with. It is my reality and I know why it exists. I have accepted the fact that every time the dishwasher flashes up digits showing me when the dishes will be clean, I will think: "hypoglycemia." I allow myself an association with boiled corn, Danai's lunch before we visited her pediatrician that Monday afternoon. As anxiety deformed the familiar features of the doctor's face, he wanted to know what Danai had eaten for lunch; in those moments, we passed from a carefree existence to a life with diabetes. I have learned to live with such experiences without being frightened. I accept them as a natural outcome of what has gone before.

After living for five years by the laws of type one diabetes and surviving a number of mental conflicts and battles, I have come to accept that I cannot face every aspect of this condition with courage. This was evident on several occasions when diabetes intensively occupied my life and I was mostly and constantly engaged in monitoring its pace. During these times, I had moments when I felt weak, as if I could not tolerate any more pressure. I knew I had reached a point when the pressure threatened my ability to maintain the balance I needed to function. I reached a point of saturation and felt that I might go beyond my limits—or even that I had already done so.

Now, when this happens, I know that I have to find ways to protect myself without guilt or procrastination. I try to put a big STOP sign in front of myself, as if I were driving a car. It isn't enough to brake; I also have to pull the hand brake and take time out, like basketball players do. By distancing myself and taking the opportunity to recharge, I can help not only myself but also my family avoid an unpleasant situation. For survival, I still have to carry out tasks that cannot be postponed. At the same time, I remain aware of the messages my body and psyche are sending me. When these are signs of exhaustion, I take them seriously and immediately seek relaxation.

For my own survival, I make sure to give my own body and mind moments to relieve pressure and unwind. When under enormous stress, I either isolate myself or become immersed in another activity, depending on my needs at that specific moment. I take walks in the forest, watch movies, drink tea while reading a book, listen to loud music, sleep, and have pleasant discussions, to mention only a few options. Such activities create a refuge. After five years with diabetes, I am more aware of things taking place around me. I enjoy the wonderful singing of birds more than I ever did before. I appreciate the sight of a small, winged being hopping in search of food. The tensions of the past five years enable me to lose myself in the wonderful colors of the sky, as the sun moves on to other neighborhoods, to wake up other diabetic children and their parents. I often imagine its rays warming other bodies in countries far away, where diabetes hurts families just as much. Five years after the first diagnosis, I can feel with greater intensity and grace the healing power of absolute peace, inaction, and meditation on body and soul.

These opportunities of escaping pressure transform me. They enable me to teach myself to focus on the happy aspects of life, and to realize that they are not self-evident and should not be taken for granted, because nothing is self-evident or able to be taken for granted. This combination of action and inaction is different from the way I lived in the past and could live in the future. It is a mixture that suits the way I feel now and satisfies present needs. It liberates my energy and helps it flow, while increasing my creativity. It keeps me psychologically balanced, and therefore I consider it an essential element of my existence.

Over time, I realized that to survive and achieve a good symbiosis with my child's diagnosis of diabetes, I would have to lower my expectations and demand less of myself. I realized that I would not be able to carry all this weight on my shoulders alone; others had to provide necessary help. So, for example, my husband almost always measures Danai´s blood sugar levels at night, because interrupted sleep does not cause him sleeping disorders, as it does me. Regardless of how much help I receive from others, I have to work on my inner world alone, through my own intentions, willpower, and initiative. Five years after the diagnosis, I know that my only real and faithful ally remains myself.

30. HOW DIABETICS LEARN: DANAI FIVE YEARS AFTER THE DIAGNOSIS.

Diabetic children learn valuable lessons from a tough and demanding teacher who is permanently in their lives. I have repeatedly mentioned the importance of regarding difficulties as more than just a negative element of life. Every effort to learn, no matter what one learns, equips one with a more flexible way of thinking and helps widen one's horizons. By coexisting with diabetes, under the right sort of guidance from trusted people, a child can discover sides of himself or herself that lead toward a new awareness.

Without intending to portray the life of the diabetic child as ideal, an in-depth look at this kind of life reveals that all the pains, insecurities, weaknesses, and problems diabetic children endure do sensitize them, bestowing an ability to walk through life alert and noticing, with sensitive feelers. Type one diabetic children, who have to work harder than others to survive, learn to care not only about their own needs, but also about the needs of those around them. I know type one diabetics who have become doctors; I assume that their early experiences awoke a need to serve other human beings. I recently read about experts in the United States of America who were working to create an artificial pancreas. The son of one of these experts was a type one diabetic child.

It is particularly rewarding for a diabetic child to feel optimistic and to realize that life offers plenty of opportunities to create, and contribute in a positive way, not just to the functioning of his or her own society, but to the whole planet. I see how much Danai's awareness has increased during the past five years. Through her condition, she has become more sensitized to the needs and problems of other people than most non-diabetic children her age. She fills up her time in a creative way giving her condition a secondary status.

I feel that Danai does not let her condition defeat her. She is strong physically as well as mentally. Her mental strength is increasing with the accumulation of positive experiences, despite the permanence of her strict teacher, diabetes. She is learning that in life you must give as well as receive. She has learned to be sensitive to other people´s problems and needs, especially children in other parts of the planet who are experiencing inconceivable difficulties and need our help. Recently, she took part in a Red Cross initiative to reunify a girl with her mother. She has learned to offer material goods to children in need, and to feel the joy of such an act.

Danai´s picture has appeared in our local paper more than once, for various reasons: once, she and Ioli were out on the street in our town collecting money for tsunami victims in Japan; another time, Danai, Ioli, and I were protesting against the cutting down of beautiful trees in our local park. Two years ago, our local newspaper published an article about Danai winning a school competition in reading unknown French texts. I cried with joy when she ran to show me the cup she had won in that competition. We fell into each other´s arms and I am sure we could have lit up a dark room with the energy our joy produced.

The same happened when she came home with another cup, this time for winning a competition in English. This thirteen-year-old diabetic also won a drawing competition; after a short break, she started dancing lessons again, this time to learn hip hop. She took a course in babysitting so that she could earn money caring for children. The positive outcome of such a life attitude is that diabetes loses its power. Danai enjoys her life, despite always holding hands with her condition.

Most of the time, she faces diabetes and its hardships with exemplary maturity, patience and responsibility, something that makes her largely independent of her father and me. This thirteen-year-old girl has earned the freedom to vary and change her daily routine, through the capable, intelligent way she manages her condition and life in general. I trust that she will go through life with confidence, despite the demands she must face on a daily basis. I expect my daughter to respect herself for all that she is, and to want to protect herself at every stage of life. Danai is taking large steps towards the future, and spreading her wings more and more towards becoming completely independent. A month ago, on her own initiative, she got her first job delivering newspapers; one of her wishes materialized very fast. She intends to save the money in her own account and invest it in driving lessons, in order to take a further step towards adulthood.

Five years after the diagnosis, diabetes does not interfere with Danai's social life. She spends more and more time with friends, shopping and going to movies and parties. With the help of the pump, she has been able to begin sleeping over at her friends' houses and regaining the freedom she lost after her diagnosis. Her friends accept the condition as part of Danai and try to be helpful in any way they can.

During the past five years, diabetes has not impeded either Danai's excellent school performance or her achievement in sports. Using the insulin pump has made it easier for her to participate in sports. During intense physical activity, she makes sure that the appropriate amount of insulin will be pumped into her body for the right amount of time in order to decrease the possibility of becoming hypoglycemic and avoid the unpleasant consequences of such a state.

Danai and I have reached the stage where she is the one encouraging me to get out of the house—to get to my appointments and pursue personal interests. This would have been inconceivable when we first started living with diabetes—I thought she would be constantly dependent on my help. By contrast, when I'm out, she prepares dinner herself, especially green salads, which she enjoys eating in front of the TV, while watching her favorite series with Ioli. She bakes gluten-free cakes and muffins, not only when she is invited to parties (where the other children's moms always provide gluten-free products), but also because she enjoys variety in her life, which she lives to the full.

Danai receives the kind of help she needs as and when she needs it. Sometimes she asks my opinion on how to regulate her diabetes. At such times, we don't need long discussions—we communicate through the briefest exchange of words. Although I want her to know that she will never be alone with diabetes, I also trust her to make the right decisions.

Some years ago, I attended a conference on diabetes in Germany. One of the other participants admitted to me that he had made a mistake when his now adult daughter was a child. When he came home from work every day, the first thing he wanted to know was how her diabetes had been. He was so worried about his daughter's health that he forgot to ask about other things, not related to diabetes, but to life in general. It did not occur to him that he could simply press the button on his daughter's measuring equipment and get the information he wanted without disrupting their relationship.

From the day we left the hospital with type one diabetes in our lives, we applied the doctor's advice without exceptions. We do not give diabetes the chance to dominate our lives, no matter how hard it tries. Danai and I prefer to talk about her day in school, what happened in class, what her friends told her, and how she or other children feel. We like to talk about the bigger and smaller events of life, about the sweetness of our pets, about politics and social phenomena, about the immense value of sincere relationships, about the stupid mistakes human beings make, about Kate and William, and even about their baby George.

The child I adore loves to tousle my hair, and to squeeze and kiss me while I'm working at my computer. She bursts into laughter when she swivels me around in my chair, while I am trying to write down these adventures. She makes me laugh when we brush our teeth standing next to each other and she swings her hips and bumps me, forgetting about her insulin pump. This thirteen-year-old girl is a normal teenager. There are moments when I get on her nerves and she gets on mine. At the same time, we both feel that the nucleus of our relationship is based on immense and authentic unconditional love, which holds us in the more than precious, sacred relationship between mother and child.

Danai is in charge of her body and she knows it. She is the captain of her own boat, always learning to move forward faster to the nicer parts of life, even after a hypoglycemic incident. One night, after measuring her sugar levels, she came into my office and just said, "42," while squeezing her cheek against mine, with lots of love and a sense of humor. I asked whether she had had any juice, and we laughingly walked to the kitchen. I told her that if she was still in such a good mood, even though her sleep had been interrupted and she'd had to leave her warm bed to deal with a hypoglycemic state, we were a strong team and nothing could affect us. On that night, Danai returned to bed in the same cheerful mood, proving how much she had learned over the years, and how strong she had become, while facing the permanent challenges her condition imposed on her.

Of course, no diabetic child can constantly demonstrate this attitude. When she feels discouraged, Danai knows that she is not alone with diabetes. At moments like these, she knows that we share the load. When she was eight years old and first diagnosed, hiding under her hospital blankets, I promised that she would never be alone with diabetes. Five years later, she knows that she can count on her parents to always be there for her, because we live in the world of diabetes together.

31. THE OTHER CHILD OF THE FAMILY: IOLI

Today, Ioli is ten, and able to explain to anyone who is interested exactly what it means to be type one diabetic. After Danai, two more children were diagnosed with type one diabetes at school, and one of them was in Ioli´s class. Her teacher asked her to talk to the other children in the class about diabetes, drawing on her experiences as Danai's sister. Despite her brilliance and willingness to help, Ioli knows that she should not feel in any way responsible for her sister´s condition. Instead, I try to help her see that she is an individual with her own needs, interests, and talents.

To meet Ioli's needs, I try to use every opportunity to do something special with her, showing that she is just as precious to me as Danai. It is important for her to have the chance to take a break from the many "musts" and "don'ts" that are indirectly imposed on her. The two of us occasionally escape to our favorite café, go to the movies, eat ice cream, cycle, and flick through books in our favorite bookshop. I want Ioli to know that this time is our time, beautiful and precious moments that are exclusively ours and absolutely essential.

My younger daughter takes piano lessons at the music school in our area and enjoys practicing, especially when she is preparing for a concert in front of a small audience. She recently transferred from primary to high school (in Germany, primary school lasts four years), where she is a member of the school choir. She is gentle and loving to our tomcats, and on rare occasions when all the planets in the universe are aligned with Earth, she even helps me clean her room. I always make a point of encouraging her to be aware of her own needs and to pursue her own interests. Although Ioli is a strong character, she still needs support and care; it is important that she not feel carried away in the swirl of diabetes and forgotten by her family. Non-diabetic children in the family also learn important life lessons. I believe that we will see the results of these when Ioli is an adult looking back on her childhood. At the moment, she hopes to start horseback riding again.

32. DIABETIC DINOSAURS: THE UNKNOWN WORLD OF DIABETES

It is my impression that diabetic children often develop stronger mental reserves than non-diabetic children, especially when they have the support and assistance of trusted adults. These reserves enable them to deal with the demands of a condition they face on a daily basis. The diabetic child is confronted with the constant need to endure, tolerate, and learn to accept strict rules and restrictions, and to live with demanding conditions that non-diabetics never experience. The fact that diabetes type one is an invisible condition makes it more difficult for non-diabetics to understand and show empathy, something that can put additional pressure on a diabetic child.

It is common knowledge that there are millions of type one diabetics worldwide. If I were to ask my readers how many of them had ever seen a diabetic inject insulin in public, I doubt that many hands would be raised. I myself have never seen anyone inject insulin in public; only once did I ever prepare a syringe for Danai in front of strangers, at a German airport. The police patrol approached and discreetly followed my movements with their eyes, as I cleared bubbles out of the syringe. I did not want to provoke them, but it was also an opportunity to teach my daughter not to feel ashamed of herself for being diabetic and not be afraid to admit her condition. On the contrary, she needs to know that it is not wrong to care for herself, no matter where she is. Right there at the airport I also had a chance to educate passersby. I hope that everyone who saw us realized that people living with different circumstances have the right to inhabit this planet, just like everybody else. I want people to know that it is neither surreal nor threatening for a diabetic to inject insulin in public.

Diabetic families also need the opportunity and incentive to talk and be heard, to teach the societies they live in and sensitize others to the peculiarities of life with type one diabetes. Such initiatives could reduce fear on both sides: on the diabetics' side, the fear of marginalization and rejection, and on the non-diabetics' side, the fear experienced when witnessing a diabetic injecting insulin.

At this point I would like to mention the comment of a non-diabetic Canadian friend, in order to demonstrate how inadequate knowledge about diabetes affects the general public, as well as diabetic families. This well-meaning friend's response to an email of family news made me realize how amazingly little people know about diabetes type one. I mentioned, among other things, that Danai had changed to an insulin pump. His message made clear that, although he lives in a country with a very high standard of living and millions of diabetics, he was unfamiliar with the world of type one diabetes and in particular with the function of the insulin pump. Although he was aware that Danai was diabetic, he had never realized that her condition was "so serious" as to require an insulin pump! He also commented that he could not imagine having a piece of artificial equipment attached to his body. Our Canadian friend's message made me smile—I knew he did not, for a moment, mean to hurt us in any way with those remarks. I mention this exchange only because our friend was a typical representative of Western society, which lacks in-depth knowledge of type one diabetes.

It is tragic, I feel, that although there are millions of type one diabetics around the world, we only occasionally hear about diabetes—for a few seconds, perhaps, on a news report. Why do most people only know that diabetics are not supposed to eat sweets? Why are issues relating to this condition only mentioned by companies selling pharmaceutical products? We often hear about the thousands of new cases of type one diabetes being diagnosed around the world every year; at the same time diabetics seem to have no presence in society. Where and under what circumstances do all these people live? Isn't their daily struggle worth understanding? In the non-diabetic world, why on earth do diabetics seem practically as extinct as dinosaurs?

Have we really reached the point of measuring quality of life by how expensive a person's mobile phone is, rather than making any effort to comprehend and accept human differences? Many smokers still feel free to light cigarettes in public, without any shame or inhibition about this harmful behavior. At the same time, diabetics feel the need to hide; they feel ashamed of their condition and afraid of being judged and commented on when they inject insulin in front of non-diabetics, even though this act is essential for their own health. To allay panic and fear, professionals of all specialties worldwide, from doctors, therapists, and nurses to anyone who works with type one diabetic children and their families, should make a sincere effort to educate non-diabetics about the kind of life diabetics lead. Their contribution could be vital in creating a more harmonious world for all of us to live in.

A world in which type one diabetics never felt the need to hide their diabetes would be a leap forward for humanity. In such a world, diabetics would not have to isolate themselves to care for their special needs, but could inject insulin wherever they were, in airports, on trains and beaches, in offices, taverns, and factories, and wherever non-diabetics congregate.

33. MY LAST THOUGHTS

Five years after my child was diagnosed with type one diabetes, I no longer feel defeated or in pain. When your own child is diagnosed with a chronic condition, there are no winners or losers. You give something and you take something in return. Today, I listen carefully to what diabetes has to say and I never stop being hopeful. I hope that one day, someone will come and shake me or wake me up, shouting with joy that a cure for type one diabetes has been found. I have read on the Internet that an enzyme or vaccine could be used to treat celiac disease in the future. I continue to hope that the suffering type one diabetics still experience will not last forever, and that one of the many researchers working feverishly to solve the riddle of type one diabetes in laboratories around the world will one day crack the code. It is a challenge similar to the one I gave Danai when we were playing hangman in the pediatrician's office five years ago, on our last day before we entered the world of diabetes type one. Until a cure is found, I will continue to love diabetes because it is part of my child.

ABOUT THE AUTHOR

Despina Margiori was born and raised in Athens, Greece. She studied Sociology at the American College of Greece (Deree College), Industrial Relations at Warwick University in England, and after working for various companies in Greece and for the Tourist Information Office of Oxford, she followed her big dream and studied Psychology at the universities TU Berlin and Justus Liebig Universität, Giessen in Germany. She is always grateful when she is given the opportunity to travel to new countries and get to know different people and learn from them. She absolutely believes in the beneficial value of volunteerism, while she will never forget her experience as a volunteer at the Olympic Games in Athens. She equally enjoys the absolute tranquility of a forest and the loud music while driving. Tennis, and everything around it, give her strength and pleasure. She has six children, four of them four legged. She lives in Germany with her family.